HORMONE REPLACEMENT THERAPY

by

R. Don Gambrell, Jr., M.D.
Clinical Professor
Department of Obstetrics and Gynecology
and Physiology and Endocrinology
Medical College of Georgia
Augusta, GA 30912-3395

Fifth Edition

EMIS, Inc.
Medical Publishers
P.O. Box 1607
Durant, OK 74702-1607

For Direct Mail Orders, write:

EMIS, Inc.
Medical Publishers
P.O. Box 1607
Durant, OK 74702-1607

Phone Orders
1-800-225-0694
FAX Orders
405-924-9414

ISBN: 0-929240-81-2

FIFTH EDITION

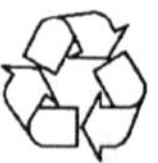

Printed on recycled paper

Published in the United States 1997

OTHER CENTER INDEX PUBLICATIONS

REPRODUCTIVE HEALTH

Breastfeeding: A Problem-Solving Manual, 4th ed. — Carroll,Saunders, & Johnson

Contraceptive Surgery for Men and Women, 2nd ed. — Moss/AVSC

Endometriosis: The Enigmatic Disease — Corson

Estrogen Replacement Therapy User Guide, 2nd ed. — Gambrell

Gynecological Care Manual for HIV Positive Women — Denenberg

Management of Infertility: A Clinician's Manual, 2nd ed. — Cohen

Managing Contraceptive Pill Patients, 8th ed. — Dickey

Managing Danazol Patients, 2nd ed. — Dickey

Menopause: Clinical Concepts, 2nd ed. — Chihal & London

Oral Contraceptive User Guide, 2nd ed. — Dickey

Safe Sex: A Guide to Condoms, 2nd ed. — Brackett

CARDIOLOGY

Cholesterol Treatment: A Guide to Lipid Disorder Management, 3rd ed. — Leaf

Emergency Cardiac Maneuvers, 2nd ed. — Bartecchi

Hypertension Treatment User Guide, 2nd ed. — Kaplan

Management of Heart Failure — Cohn & Kubo

Management of Hypertension, 6th ed. — Kaplan

GENERAL MEDICINE

A Manual on Drug Dependence — Nahas

A Practical Anesthesia Information Guide — Jerome

Arthritis Therapy: A Clinician's Manual — Kantor

Assessment and Management of the Suicidal Adolescent — Clayton

Breast Disease in Women and Men — Shuler

Handbook of Headache Disorders, 2nd ed. — Elkind

Management of Aneurysmal Subarachnoid Hemorrhage — Fossett

Management of Diabetes Mellitus, 3rd ed. — Schwartz

Medical Management of Depression — DeBattista & Glick

Mid-Life Sexuality: Enrichment and Problem-Solving — Semmens

Projective Psychodiagnostic Assessment — Caldwell & Dixon

Primary Mental Health Care — Berman*

EDUCATION

Chief Executive Officer's Guide For Health Facility Development, 2nd ed. — Weeks

Children with Special Needs, 2nd ed. — Bradway & Block

Infection Prevention for Family Planning Service Programs — Tietjen, Cronin & McIntosh (JHPIEGO)*

Resilience Enhancement for the Resident Physician — Messner*

Travel Well: A Gourmet Guide to Healthy Travel — Kaplan*

**Not Center-Indexed Publications*

DEDICATION

This book is dedicated to my wife, Caroline, who for more than 40 years has supported my every endeavor with love, warmth, and kind understanding.

NOTES

TABLE OF CONTENTS

TABLES

FIGURES

#1 Introduction

Menopausal Hormone Deficiency

After the menopause, the average woman still has one-third of her lifespan ahead. However, women's experience of the menopause and its effects on their remaining years vary widely (see Figure 1.1).

The declining ovarian function can be rapid for some and slower for others. Some women may produce sufficient endogenous estrogens to remain asymptomatic, but others develop a variety of disturbances during the climacteric, a term in current use for the premenopausal, menopausal, and postmenopausal period.

These symptoms may include:

- Hot flushes (or flashes)
- Night sweats
- Vaginal irritation or dryness
- Insomnia
- Depression

The issue of what should be done about adverse climacteric symptoms is controversial. There is general agreement that menopause is a hormone-deficient state and should be treated. Physicians are now asking what dosages of estrogen should be used and what regimens of hormone replacement are best for their patients.

No longer is it contended that menopausal symptoms are psychoneurotic. It is no longer thought that only vasomotor manifestations (hot flushes, sweats) and atrophic vaginitis are directly due to the estrogen deficit and that these manifestations may be treated with a smallest possible dose of oral estrogens for a short period of time.

Trends in Treatment

Estrogen replacement therapy is controversial. It was fashionable in the 1960s, but in the 1970s complications became apparent. Physicians became reluctant to treat the climacteric, and patients became wary of hormone therapy because of widely publicized reports that estrogens cause endometrial cancer. In the 1980s, however, hormone therapy grew in popularity, and this trend is continuing into the 1990s.

First, there has been a growing recognition of the dangers of long-term estrogen deficiency, which can lead to development of:

- Osteoporosis
- Atherosclerotic heart disease
- Psychogenic manifestations
- Alzheimer's disease

Although it has not been directly shown that estrogen deficiency increases the risk for colon cancer, several new studies have observed that therapy with any sex steroid (estrogen, progestogen, or androgen) decreases the risk for colon cancer (see Section #12).

There is growing acknowledgment that estrogen deficiency should be treated as vigorously as any other endocrinopathy and without a necessary limitation of time. Instead of the minimal treatments suggested in the past to alleviate specific symptoms, some women require hormonal therapy:

- For years instead of months
- Continuously instead of cyclically
- In larger dosages than were previously recommended

Further, there is a recognition that some postmenopausal women need treatment with other hormones (e.g., progestogen) to prevent endometrial hyperplasia and subsequent neoplasia.

Second, the belief that estrogen treatment causes endometrial cancer is no longer valid. The incidence of cancer of the endometrium or of the breast need not increase as a result of long-term estrogen therapy if cyclic progestogens in adequate dosages are added to the estrogen regimen.

FIGURE 1.1 - Age of Menopause

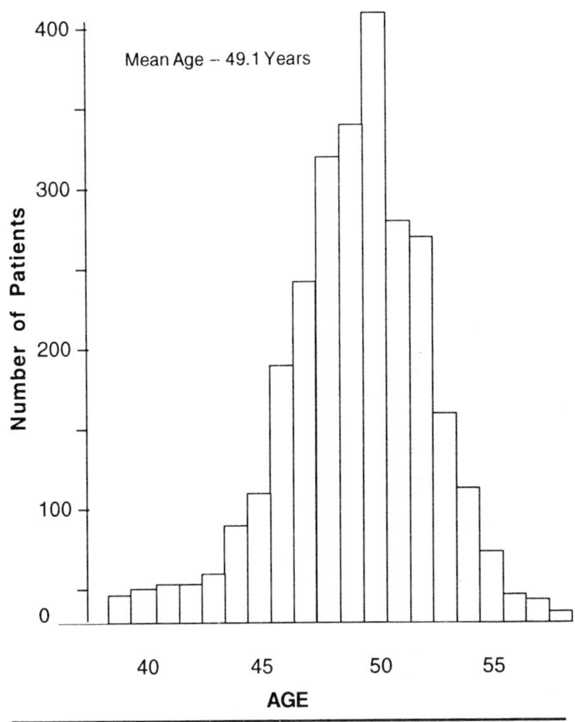

The age of menopause in more than 2,000 women undergoing natural menopause. (Reproduced with permission of the publisher; the American Fertility Society, from Gambrell) (Ref 54).

Clinical Information

Most women who seek medical attention for menopausal symptoms complain of vasomotor symptoms. These include:

- Hot flushes (or flashes)
- Night sweats

These symptoms usually:

- Have an insidious onset
- Increase as serum estrogens decline
- Are variable in frequency and severity
- May persist for several months to a few years

Research

Studies have shown an association between the pulsatile release of LH and the occurrence of hot flushes. However, LH levels in and of themselves are not responsible for triggering vasomotor symptoms, since these phenomena can occur after hypophysectomy. If untreated, the hypothalamus and autonomic nervous systems gradually adjust to the lower levels of estrogen and eventually hot flushes abate.

Patients with gonadal dysgenesis have high levels of gonadotropins. However, these individuals experience vasomotor symptoms only after exposure to exogenous estrogens and subsequent withdrawal.

Recommendations

In the past, low dosages of estrogen have been given for short intervals and then reduced gradually so that hot flushes fade. This concept is no longer valid. A woman experiencing menopausal symptoms has become estrogen-deficient and will remain so for the rest of her life.

A balanced program of estrogen replacement therapy combined with cyclic progestogens is the best treatment, since the real goal of estrogen replacement is not only to alleviate vasomotor symptoms but to prevent later metabolic consequences, such as osteoporosis and atherosclerosis.

#3 Urogenital Atrophy

3.

Clinical Information

Atrophy of the genital epithelium may result in senile vaginitis (Ref 15). Symptoms may include:

- Irritation
- Burning
- Pruritus
- Leukorrhea
- Dyspareunia
- Vaginal bleeding
- Decrease of vaginal secretions
- Thinning and easily-traumatized epithelium
- Shortening and lessening of distensibility of the vagina

Most sexual problems experienced by postmenopausal women are due to the physical status of the vaginal mucosa, which must maintain sufficient protective moisture and provide lubrication during coitus. After menopause, atrophic changes may lead to:

- Dyspareunia
- Vaginitis
- Vaginismus
- Physical discomfort
- Loss of sexual interest

Research

Studies have demonstrated (Ref 135) that the estrogen-deprived state in postmenopausal women leads to changes in:

- Quantity of vaginal fluid
- pH levels
- Vaginal blood flow

However, urogenital changes that develop because of estrogen deprivation are reversible with estrogen replacement therapy, although the longer the estrogen deprivation, the slower the physiologic response.

Recommendations

The preferred treatment for atrophic vaginitis is local estrogen therapy in the form of vaginal creams (e.g., Premarin and Estrace), which are well absorbed into the vaginal mucosa. Daily bedtime applications should be given for one to two weeks; thereafter, applications three times per week are normally sufficient for maintenance (see Section #14).

Systemic therapy by oral or other routes is usually started simultaneously. Local vaginal therapy can sometimes be discontinued after a few months, or continued vaginal cream treatment may be required in addition to systemic estrogens. Irritative symptoms abate rapidly with estrogen vaginal cream, but restoration of normal vaginal blood flow may take up to a year.

To a lesser extent, the vulvar epithelium also becomes thin and may be irritated or subject to infection. These conditions commonly respond to applications of vaginal estrogen cream, but a one- or two-percent testosterone cream may be necessary for kraurosis vulva or other atrophic or leukoplakic vulvar conditions. Vulvar pruritus may sometimes require one-percent hydrocortisone creams or other glucocorticoid creams for relief in addition to either estrogen or testosterone creams.

The integrity of the lower urinary tract mucosa is dependent upon estrogens. Estrogen deficiency may therefore result in irritative symptoms such as:

- Dysuria
- Burning on urination

- Cystitis
- Urethral caruncles
- Nongonococcal urethritis

These symptoms respond best to local applications of vaginal estrogen creams with the simultaneous initiation of oral estrogen therapy.

NOTES

4.

#4 Psychogenic Manifestations

Clinical Information

Many postmenopausal women complain of psychogenic disturbances. These may include:

- Increased nervousness
- Depression
- Anxiety
- Insomnia
- Headaches

Other conditions that may be aggravated by menopausal symptoms include:

- Pre-existing psychosomatic problems intensified by hot flushes
- Sleep patterns disturbed by night sweats
- Decreased libido due to atrophic vaginitis and resulting in dyspareunia

Research

Carefully controlled double-blind and crossover studies indicate that estrogens have a tonic mental effect (Ref 34). Estrogen patients had higher scores on psychometric evaluations, alleviating the psychogenic manifestations independent of vasomotor symptoms (Ref 18).

Moderate to severe depression, as measured by the Zung Self-Rating Depression Scale, was significantly higher in patients who had surgical menopause by hysterectomy with or without bilateral oophorectomy compared to women undergoing natural menopause (Ref 3). This suggests that women undergoing pelvic surgery have either not been reconciled to its necessity or were insufficiently prepared for its consequences.

In a study using pellets of estradiol, testosterone, or placebo, testosterone increased the frequency and intensity of orgasmic responses (Ref 148). In a double-blind study using hot flushes as the main index, 96 percent of patients improved on estrogens and 91 percent on an estrogen-androgen combination. Fair to good results were obtained in 56 percent of patients receiving androgens, and 16 percent of those were given a placebo. The estrogen-androgen combination was associated with less withdrawal bleeding and accentuated well-being and healthy libido (Ref 149).

Headaches in postmenopausal women are frequently regarded as psychosomatic and not hormone-related; but in one study using estrogen, progestogen, and placebo, headaches were alleviated while high levels of estrogen were maintained (Ref 34).

In a study of 85 patients receiving hormone replacement therapy when headaches were a secondary complaint, relief from headaches was obtained by the administration of estradiol pellets alone or in combination with testosterone (Ref 69).

Although these studies may not prove that psychogenic complaints of postmenopausal women are hormone-dependent, they indicate that many are hormone-responsive, since patients improve once therapy is begun.

Recommendations

Sexual dysfunction in menopausal women, long regarded by psychologists and sex therapists as psychogenic, has been shown to be responsive to hormone therapy. Relief may be afforded by:

- Estrogens, including estrogen vaginal cream, for complaints such as:
  - Vaginal dryness
  - Dyspareunia
- Androgens, for complaints of loss of sexual interest (see Section #15)

It is important to note that a postmenopausal woman who has lost up to two-thirds of estrogen production has also lost up to one-half of androgen production. Although most postmenopausal women respond well to estrogen-progestogen therapy, some require the addition of an androgen. Women treated with estrogen-androgen replacement therapy were more composed, elated, and energetic than those treated with estrogen alone (Ref 138). The addition of androgen enhanced sexual desire and increased the frequency of sexual fantasies compared to estrogen alone or with placebo. In the Yale Mid-Life Study Program, androgens are not routinely prescribed unless there is a deficiency in the total or free testosterone levels (Ref 133).

NOTES

#5 Osteoporosis

Clinical Information

Osteoporosis is a skeletal disorder primarily affecting trabecular bone in which a reduction in the quantity of bone predisposes to fracture. It is now recognized that age-related or Type II osteoporosis is also under the influence of estrogens. Hip fractures, where the bone is primarily cortical, are also prevented with estrogen therapy. Although both sexes lose bone mass with aging, it is rare for men to develop symptomatic osteoporosis before age 70.

This is a major public health problem affecting 25 million older Americans, of which 90 percent are postmenopausal women (Ref 120). Approximately 25 percent of white women older than age 60 have spinal compression fractures. This number increases to 50 percent by age 75. With increasing longevity, a woman reaching age 50 now has a life expectancy of 80.4 years, when the already serious morbidity and mortality associated with postmenopausal osteoporosis becomes even greater. Of all hip fractures, 80 percent are associated with osteoporosis; 34 percent of all elderly patients with hip fractures die within six months (Ref 68).

Research

Several studies have been conducted into the effects of estrogen therapy on the prevention of osteoporosis. These studies have demonstrated that estrogen therapy:

- Prevents osteoporosis
- Decreases vertebral, hip, and other fractures
- Prevents further loss of height

In one long-term prospective study of 1,000 women treated with estrogens for 15 years (14,318 patient-years of observation), wrist fractures were reduced by 70 percent from the expected rate (Ref 16). No hip fractures occurred during 15 years of estrogen therapy in these 1,000 women. In a carefully controlled ongoing study from the Mayo Clinic, patients treated with calcium carbonate (1,500 to 2,000 mg daily) had 419 vertebral fractures per 1,000 patient years of observation compared to 834 per 1,000 in the placebo-treated group (Ref 127). Fracture rate was reduced by 61 percent to 304 per 1,000 in those treated with calcium plus sodium fluoride (50 to 60 mg daily).

However, the most effective therapy, with a vertebral fracture rate of 53 per 1,000, was the combination of:

- Conjugated estrogens (0.625 to 2.5 mg daily)
- Sodium fluoride
- Calcium

The addition of vitamin D had no significant effect and was associated with a substantial incidence of hypercalcemia or hypercalciuria. Thus, the Mayo group did not believe that vitamin D should be included in therapy for osteoporosis.

In a later study from this group, although trabecular bone density was increased with fluoride therapy, cortical bone density was decreased, which increased skeletal fragility (Ref 128). Since this may increase the risk for hip fracture, the Mayo group has abandoned fluoride therapy, continuing the use of estrogen and calcium.

Recommendations

The recommendations of the National Institutes of Health Conference on Osteoporosis are that:

- Estrogen therapy is the best prevention and treatment of osteoporosis
- Calcium supplementation, which should be begun at about age 40 or approximately 10 years prior to menopause, should be given in dosages of 1,000 mg of elemental calcium daily (see Section #18)
- Weight-bearing exercise is the best activity to prevent osteoporosis (Ref 120)

An international consensus conference confirmed that estrogen replacement, supplemental calcium, and exercise were the mainstays in preventing osteoporosis (Ref 98). Fluoride may increase trabecular bone mass but should not be used in predominantly cortical osteoporosis; it does not have a place in the prophylaxis of bone loss. Additionally, vitamin D and anabolic steroids do not prevent osteoporosis. Calcitonin may be useful for women at high risk for whom estrogens are contraindicated (see Section #29). Cyclic and coherence therapies (ADFR) are promising but need more research.

Diphosphonates, e.g., etidronate, reduce bone loss and the incidence of vertebral deformity in patients with established postmenopausal osteoporosis (Ref 98). Etidronate's effect on nonvertebral fracture, long-term skeletal impact, and patients in whom diphosphonates are most appropriate remains to be identified. Etidronate therapy is usually administered daily for the first two weeks at three-month intervals, followed by 11 weeks of calcium supplementation only. Candidates for etidronate therapy currently include patients with radiographic evidence of spinal osteoporosis with or without fractures.

Fosamax is a newly released bisphosphonate, approved for treatment of postmenopausal osteoporosis. The dosage is 10 mg daily and must be taken before the first food of the day with a glass of water. Its principal side effect is gastrointestinal irritation. The drug shows great promise in spinal osteoporosis in that trabecular bone in the vertebrae may increase five to 10 percent over the first two years and vertebral fractures may decrease by 50 percent.

In a 3 three-year study, alendronate reduced hip fractures by 51.3 percent and wrist fractures by 47 percent. Although the 10 mg dosage is used to treat osteoporosis, 5 mg has just been approved by the FDA to prevent osteoporosis. However, estrogen replacement therapy is still preferred because of the many other benefits.

Conjugated estrogens 0.625 mg daily is the dosage of estrogen shown to prevent osteoporosis in 90 percent of postmenopausal women. Higher dosages of estrogen, e.g., 1.25 to 2.5 mg, are required if osteoporosis is already present (Ref 43, 96).

There has recently been renewed interest in estropipate (Ogen, Ortho-Est); however, it must be remembered that, milligram for milligram, this estrogen has less biologic activity than conjugated estrogens. The minimum effective dosage of estropipate that will prevent osteoporosis is 1.25 mg.

Also, a lower dosage of micronized estradiol has become available (Estrace 0.5 mg). It is unlikely that this dosage will prevent osteoporosis over the long term. In the only published dose-ranging study, patients treated with 0.5 mg micronized estradiol only maintained bone mass for 18 months, while those treated with 1 or 2 mg gained bone mass (Ref 44). When the group treated with 0.5 mg were crossed over to 1 mg for the second 18 months, they gained two percent in bone mineral content, while those who continued on 1 mg gained additional bone mass. There are no studies showing that 0.5 mg estradiol will prevent bone loss for at least three years.

Prevention

Prevention of postmenopausal osteoporosis may not be unique to estrogens, since therapy with an injectable progestogen is also effective in preventing bone loss (Ref 95). The addition of a progestogen to estrogen therapy may be important in preventing osteoporosis but may be essential in treating patients who already have osteoporosis (Ref 154).

While most studies indicate that estrogen therapy inhibits the resorption of calcium from bone (most likely by restoring calcitonin levels that are decreased after menopause), at least eight clinical studies and one good animal study have shown that combination estrogen-progestogen therapy may actually increase bone mass by promoting new bone formation.

In a 10-year double-blind prospective study, significant differences were observed between patients receiving cyclic estrogen-progestogen therapy and those given placebo (Ref 107). In women given combination estrogen-progestogen therapy less than three years after the onset of menopause, bone density increased for the entire 10 years. Although there was some bone demineralization in the estrogen-progestogen users when therapy was started later than three years after menopause, the loss of bone mass was significantly less than in either placebo group. This study emphasizes the importance of beginning estrogen-progestogen replacement early into menopause, but it also indicates that these hormones are beneficial to osteoporotic women, regardless of age. It should be noted that conjugated estrogens at 2.5 mg daily was the dosage used in this study.

In a crossover study comparing the effects of estrogen-progestogen therapy with placebo, bone mineral content increased during the three years of combination hormone therapy but continued to decline in the placebo-treated group (Figure 5.1) (Ref 22). When some patients in the estrogen-progestogen group were changed to placebo, bone density decreased. Bone mass also increased in placebo-treated women after they switched to active hormone therapy.

Another group (Ref 32) compared the effects of estrogen only to the estrogen-progestogen combination on the metabolic parameters of bone loss; these were:

- Plasma calcium
- Urinary calcium/creatinine ratio
- Hydroxyproline

All values were diminished with estrogen therapy and decreased further when a progestogen was added to the estrogen.

More recent studies indicate that hormonal therapy protects against both cervical and trochanteric hip fracture (Ref 110). Women showing the greatest such effect also had the highest proportion of treatment with estrogen and progestogen combined. Bone mineral content increased from 7.9 percent up to 28.7 percent for up to five years, even in women who did not start therapy until past age 60, when combination estrogen-progestogen therapy was used (Ref 93). Added progestogen may be particularly important for increasing cortical bone. There seems to be a synergistic effect, with lower dosages of estrogen plus progestogen having the same effect as higher dosages of estrogen (Ref 46).

The new continuous combined method of estrogen-progestogen administration has shown a net gain of 6.4 percent per year in vertebral bone density compared to 5.4 percent a year with sequential estrogen-progestogen therapy (Ref 105). The net gain in forearm bone density was similar, 3.6 percent per year with continuous and 3.7 percent per year with sequential estrogen-progestogen therapy. A recent review concluded that progesterone is active in bone metabolism, acting directly on bone by engaging in osteoblast receptor or indirectly through competition for a glucocorticoid receptor (Ref 125). Progesterone seems to promote bone formation and/or increase turnover of bone. Animal studies in oophorectomized cynomolgus monkeys indicate that trabecular bone volume was greatest in the estrogen replacement therapy plus progesterone group compared to the estrogen treatment group (Ref 82).

Is It Ever Too Late?

The concept that it is never too late to begin hormone replacement has been confirmed in a recent study of patients with established osteoporosis 14.6 ± 0.9 years from menopause (Ref 97). Previous studies have shown that fracture rate could be reduced with estrogen therapy (Ref 127) and that new bone could be formed with estrogen-progestogen therapy for 10 years (Ref 107). Estrogen therapy increased vertebral bone mass (+10.6 percent; $P \leq 0.01$) and bone density at the femoral neck (+5.5 percent; $P \leq 0.01$) (Ref 97). The group treated with 1,500 mg calcium alone lost bone at both sites. The response to estrogen was greatest in those who were furthest from menopause ($R=0.38$; $P \leq 0.05$) and among those who had the lowest bone mass ($R=-0.34$; $P \leq 0.05$).

There is no question that the best time to begin hormone therapy is at menopause to prevent osteoporosis. However, it is never too late, since bone can be restored, especially with combination estrogen-progestogen therapy.

FIGURE 5.1 - Bone Mineral Content

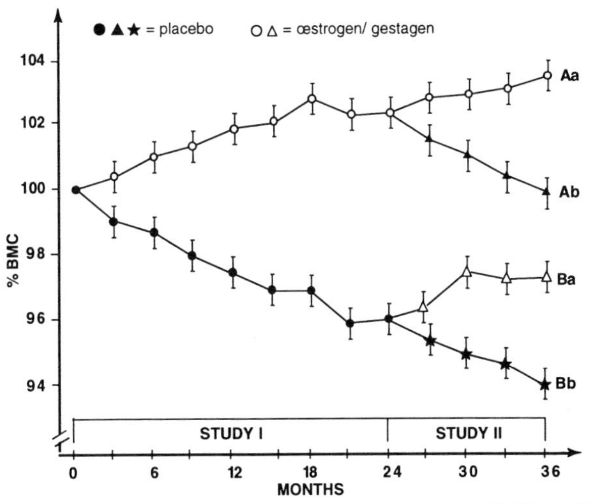

Bone mineral content as a function of time and treatment in postmenopausal women. (Reproduced with permission of the author and publisher) (Ref 22).

#6 Coronary Artery Disease

Clinical Information

Although not yet listed by the FDA as an approved indication, the greatest benefit that will accrue to postmenopausal estrogen users is prevention of coronary artery disease. More than 100 studies of all types—clinical, epidemiologic, angiographic, basic sciences, animal experimentation, and laboratory—indicate at least a 50-percent reduction in heart disease and stroke. Myocardial infarction rarely occurs in young women prior to menopause. Younger women who have had bilateral oophorectomy demonstrate a higher incidence of myocardial infarction unless estrogen therapy is begun soon after the ovaries are removed. More than 450,000 women die every year in the U.S. from heart disease and stroke; many of these deaths are preventable.

Prevention

Several studies suggest that estrogens may exert a protective effect against cardiovascular disease and stroke, especially when low dosages of natural estrogens sufficient to relieve menopausal symptoms are used. In a review of epidemiologic evidence, although all studies observed significant protection, cross-sectional and prospective external control studies observed the lowest relative risks from 0.3 to 0.4 (Ref 141). Perhaps the best studies are provided by the cohort studies with internal controls (RR=0.58; 95 percent CI, 0.48 to 0.70). A summary estimate of all studies omitting the hospital-based case control studies yielded an RR of 0.52.

The Nurses' Health Study (Ref 142) confirmed that:

- Ever estrogen use significantly reduced the risk of coronary artery disease (RR=0.5; P=0.007)
- Current estrogen use reduced the risk even lower (RR=0.3; P=0.001)
- These benefits held after adjustments for factors such as:
  - Smoking
  - Hypertension
  - Diabetes
  - High cholesterol
  - Parental history of myocardial infarction
  - Previous use of oral contraceptives
  - Obesity

Angiography Studies

At least three cardiology studies using angiography have observed less coronary artery occlusion in estrogen users (Ref 70, 103, 151). A 56- to 63-percent reduction in risk for developing severe coronary artery stenosis in women who used estrogen was observed. Sullivan et al. (Ref 151) assessed the 10-year survival rate of 2,268 menopausal women who had varying degrees of angiographically defined coronary artery atherosclerosis with respect to estrogen use. In women without demonstrable coronary artery disease at the initial angiogram, there was no statistically significant difference in the 10-year survival rate of never-users (85 percent, n=347) vs ever-users (95.6 percent, n=99). However, in women with more than 70-percent lumen stenosis at the initial angiogram, the 10-year survival rate of never-users dropped to 60 percent (n=1,108) and was significantly less than the 97-percent 10-year survival rate among ever users (n=70; P=0.027). In another study, the age-adjusted odds ratios for use of postmenopausal estrogen among women with moderate and severe levels of occlusion of coronary arteries were 0.59 (95 percent CI, 0.48 to 0.73) and 0.37 (95 percent CI, 0.29 to 0.46), respectively, which indicated a statistically significant protective effect of postmenopausal estrogen on coronary occlusion (Ref 70).

Animal Experimentation

Animal studies using cynomolgus macaque monkeys fed an atherogenic diet found that male and ovariectomized female monkeys did not differ with respect to coronary artery atherosclerosis, while premenopausal females had half the coronary artery disease of their counterparts (Ref 1). Hormone replacement therapy halved the extent of coronary artery atherosclerosis in oophorectomized monkeys compared to control animals. In delineating some of the mechanisms of coronary vessel protection, acetylcholine produced vasoconstriction of coronary arteries in postmenopausal monkeys; but when estrogen was replaced, there was coronary vasodilation. When medroxyprogesterone acetate was added to estrogen replacement therapy, there was neither vasodilation nor vasoconstriction to acetylcholine. However, there was some suggestion that monkeys treated with conjugated estrogens and medroxyprogesterone acetate had larger lumens than monkeys treated with estrogen alone.

Estrogen use also reduces the risk of cerebrovascular disease, but this has not been observed in every study. In the study that used the general population as a comparison group, there was a significantly decreased risk of stroke (RR=0.54; 95 percent CI, 0.24 to 0.84) (Ref 81). In the four prospective studies using internal controls, all found estrogen use to be beneficial, with RRs ranging from 0.23 to 0.63 (Ref 2, 75, 76, 117, 122). Both the Nurses' Health

Study and the Framingham Study failed to find decreased risk of stroke in estrogen users (Ref 142, 161). In the Leisure World Study, protection from stroke was observed in all age groups except the youngest (RR=0.53; 95 percent CI, 0.31 to 0.91) (Ref 117). This decreased risk was unaltered by adjustments for possible confounding variables such as:

- Smoking
- Alcohol
- Body mass
- Exercise

Direct Effects of Estrogen

Although from 25 to 50 percent of the effective effect of estrogen on cardiovascular disease is mediated through improved lipid patterns, there are also direct effects (Ref 132), such as:

- Estrogen and progesterone receptors identified in coronary vessel walls
- Improved vascular blood flow
- Dilation of coronary arteries
- Increased EDRF (endothelial-derived relaxing factor)
- Reduced vascular resistance
- Increased velocity of blood flow
- Increased cardiac output
- Inhibited atherosclerosis progression
- Decreased platelet adhesiveness
- Inhibited coronary thrombosis
- Prostacyclin and thromboxane metabolism
- Peripheral vasodilation

#7 Alzheimer's Disease

Clinical Information

There is considerable evidence that estrogen has an effect on the central nervous system (CNS). Estrogen deficiency may contribute to the neurodegenerative changes of the aging CNS and increase the incidence of senile dementia of the Alzheimer's type. The incidence of Alzheimer's disease increases more in women than in men after age 65, so that age-specific rates vary from 1.5 to 3.0 times that of men (Ref 12).

Research

Two of the many findings in Alzheimer's disease are a decrease in dendritic spines and a deficiency of the cholinesterase enzymes necessary to reconvert the neurotransmitters to acetyl choline. Studies in oophorectomized animals indicate that axonal and/or dendritic growth of cholinergic neurons and acetyl cholinesterase processes increased in the estrogen-treated animals, while in controls, the acetyl cholinesterase reaction was essentially localized only on cell bodies (Ref 78). These cholinergic nuclei in the brain are involved in most memory functions, and this population of cells undergoes the most pronounced degenerative changes seen in Alzheimer's disease.

Some but not all clinical studies have observed that estrogen therapy improves cognitive function. In a study of 65-year-old women, estrogen users had significantly higher scores on short- and long-term verbal memory tasks compared to women who had never used estrogen (Ref 87). However, no differences were found between estrogen users and nonusers on measures of visual/spatial memory.

In a Japanese study of seven women with Alzheimer's disease, six showed improvement in dementia ($P \leq 0.05$) (Ref 77). In a study of women with dementia, none of the 158 cases were currently using estrogen, whereas 15 percent of the matched controls were (Ref 12). The resulting relative risk of dementia in women taking estrogens was RR=0.07 ($P \leq 0.001$).

The Leisure World studies observed a 30-percent reduction of Alzheimer's disease in estrogen users (Ref 116). In a study of 2,529 female cohort members who died, the risk of Alzheimer's disease and related dementia was less in estrogen users compared to nonusers (RR=0.69; 95 percent CI, 0.46 to 1.03). The risk decreased significantly with increasing estrogen dosage and duration of use.

A large prospective study of 1,124 elderly women indicated that the age of onset of Alzheimer's disease was significantly later in women who had taken estrogen than in those who had not (RR=0.4; 95 percent CI, 0.22 to 0.85) (Ref 152).

Another epidemiologic study did not observe any reduction in Alzheimer's disease with estrogen use (Ref 14).

In a study of 107 female Alzheimer's disease cases, the RR was 1.1 (95 percent CI, 0.6 to 1.8). However, this study only evaluated ever estrogen use, including vaginal estrogen cream, while the Leisure World study observed the greatest decrease with increasing estrogen dosage and duration of use.

It appears that the latest benefit of hormone replacement therapy will be a decreased incidence of Alzheimer's disease.

#8 Vaginal Hormonal Cytology

Clinical Information

A patient's complaints of menopausal symptoms may be sufficient reason to begin estrogen replacement therapy (see Section #1). However, the vaginal smear is a good reflection of endogenous estrogen production.

With normal endogenous estrogen, there should be a high percentage (15 to 30 percent) of superficial cells (cells with small pyknotic nuclei and a large amount of cytoplasm) and the remaining cells should be of the intermediate types (larger nuclei with the nucleolus visible but still mostly cytoplasm). When parabasal cells (with a nucleus-to-cytoplasmic ratio of 50:50 or greater) are present on the vaginal smear, the patient usually has decreased estrogen production. If the vaginal smear is comprised of more than 50-percent parabasal cells, the patient is in a very hypoestrogenic state.

The physician can prepare the smear and read the vaginal hormonal cytology personally in order to provide instant information or send the vaginal smear to a cytology or pathology lab for a report of the maturation index (the percentage of superficial, intermediate, and parabasal cells). Most Pap smear reports now list an estrogen index.

Cytology Procedure

The smear is best taken from the lateral vaginal wall because it is usually more free of mucus and debris. A good instant stain for vaginal hormonal cytology is one-percent pinacyanol. The pinacyanol chloride powder dye is obtained from the Eastman Kodak Company, and the solution is made with one gram of dye in 100 cc of 90- to 95-percent alcohol (either ethanol or methanol).

After smearing the vaginal mucosa cells on a glass slide, a few drops of pinacyanol are applied and allowed to dry for one minute, then rinsed with ordinary tap water. Slides are long-lasting, and the purple color can be freshened with drops of water or oil.

Fern Pattern Procedure

Another simple test used for estimation of estrogen production is the fern pattern of cervical mucus, although this can only be used with patients who have not had hysterectomies.

Mucus from the cervix is smeared onto a glass slide and allowed to dry for five minutes. If the fern pattern appears under the microscope, normal estrogen production is indicated, since the salts only crystallize with estrogen unopposed by progesterone.

During the normal ovulatory cycle, the fern pattern of cervical mucus increases from menses until ovulation and then rapidly disappears after ovulation due to progesterone. The fern pattern is also absent during pregnancy even though estrogen levels are high, because the high progesterone levels keep the cervical mucus from ferning.

Summary

Vaginal hormonal cytology and cervical mucus fern pattern cannot be used to diagnose menopause or to follow the effects of estrogen therapy, but these are adjunctive simple methods useful in evaluating patients with menopausal symptoms.

Estrogen replacement therapy should not be denied to severely symptomatic women on the basis of what appears to be a normal estrogen smear. Consideration should also be given to initiating hormone replacement in asymptomatic postmenopausal women with very hypoestrogenic vaginal smears. The latter group would possibly benefit from additional testing for osteoporosis risk by dual x-ray absorptiometry (DXA).

Most symptomatic postmenopausal women need no additional testing other than the simple measures outlined above and the basic routine tests (see Section #12).

NOTES

#9 Progestogen Challenge Test

Clinical Information

The progestogen challenge test should be administered to all postmenopausal women with intact uteri at annual evaluation. Included in this group are:

- Symptomatic women being evaluated for estrogen replacement therapy
- Estrogen-treated patients not already on progestogen therapy
- Asymptomatic postmenopausal women

The progesterone challenge test is the most reliable test for assessing potential estrogenic stimulation of the endometrium.

Not all postmenopausal women need estrogen replacement therapy, since many produce sufficient endogenous estrogens to remain asymptomatic and prevent the metabolic changes of estrogen deficiency in later life, such as:

9.

- Atrophic vaginitis
- Osteoporosis
- Atherosclerosis

However, within this group may be those in greatest need of cyclic progestogen therapy to prevent endometrial hyperplasia (which may lead to adenocarcinoma).

Research

The progestogen challenge test was a concept evolved at Wilford Hall USAF Medical Center when it was recognized that the second highest incidence of endometrial cancer was observed in untreated postmenopausal women (Ref 50, 55, 61).

Original work on the progestogen challenge test has been confirmed by a prospective study using 100 mg of progesterone in oil given intramuscularly (Ref 74). In a study of 30 asymptomatic postmenopausal women, five had withdrawal bleeding to the progestogen challenge and three of these (60 percent) had either adenomatous or atypical adenomatous hyperplasia. In the 25 subjects with no withdrawal bleeding, the endometrial histology was normal, mostly atrophic or inactive endometrium. There were no adenocarcinomas in either group; and, although the number of subjects was small, the difference between the two groups was statistically significant ($P \leq 0.001$).

In the second phase of this study in which 10 patients with known adenomatous hyperplasia were tested, the progestogen challenge test resulted in withdrawal bleeding in nine (90 percent), confirming the effectiveness of this test in detecting abnormal endometrial pathology.

The conclusion was that the progestogen challenge test was a reliable screening test for detecting women at greater risk for developing endometrial hyperplasia or adenocarcinoma. Other studies have confirmed that the progestogen challenge test is a reliable test for identifying women at high risk for endometrial cancer (Ref 41).

In a study in which the progestogen challenge test was given to 292 elderly women (mean age = 71.2 years), 14 (4.8 percent) had either spotting or bleeding (Ref 123). Endometrial biopsies revealed significant pathology in three of these women: one endometrial cancer, one hyperplasia, and one chronic endometritis. Atrophic endometrium was found in eight, a proliferative endometrium in one, and an insufficient sample in two.

Procedure

The progestogen challenge test is performed by administering a 13-day course of progestogen (either Provera 10 mg or Aygestin 5 mg) to postmenopausal women with intact uteri (see Section #16). If a positive response occurs, as manifested by withdrawal bleeding, progestogens should be continued for 13 days each month for as long as withdrawal bleeding follows. If there is a negative response, it is recommended that the progestogen challenge be repeated each year in asymptomatic postmenopausal women not taking hormones.

Annual endometrial biopsies are not necessary in estrogen-progestogen users (see Section #10). Because of the benefits of added progestogen on the bones and the breast (see Sections #5 and #21), this hormone should be continued in estrogen users, regardless of withdrawal bleeding.

NOTES

#10 Endometrial Biopsy

Clinical Information

Women receiving unopposed estrogen therapy should have annual endometrial biopsies. Postmenopausal women with any abnormal bleeding or responding by bleeding to the progestogen challenge test should have one of the following:

- An extensive endometrial biopsy
- Clinic curettage
- Formal diagnostic dilatation and curettage (D&C)

Perimenopausal women who have irregular menses should have each of the following:

- Extensive endometrial sampling
- Pap smear
- Cervical biopsy, after Schiller's stain or colposcopically-directed
- Endocervical curettage
- Bimanual examination

10. An exception to these in estrogen-progestogen users is in situations in which bleeding occurs on or after day 11 of progestogen therapy; in these cases, no evaluation is necessary since the histology has been shown to be predominantly secretory (Ref 115). Because of the recent appearance of several cases of endometrial cancer after years of amenorrhea in patients using continuous combined estrogen-progestogen therapy, any spotting or breakthrough bleeding after the first year of therapy should be promptly investigated (see Section #20).

Endometrial Evaluation Methods

The traditional method for evaluating the endometrium has been diagnostic D&C. However, hospitalization for a D&C (even on an outpatient basis) has disadvantages, including:

- Increased anesthetic risk
- Additional expense
- Delay in diagnosis

These problems can be avoided by a properly performed clinic or office curettage, performed by carefully using the Pipelle Endometrial Suction Curette. The endometrial cavity should be sampled twice if much tissue is extracted. Frequently, the endometrial Pipelle can be utilized without a tenaculum or without sounding the uterus. This process will yield as much information as a hospital D&C.

Although there is patient discomfort with the office procedure, the discomfort may be minimized by gentleness and a careful explanation of each step. Discomfort can also be reduced by placing four-percent Xylocaine Viscous on a small cotton-tipped applicator in the endocervical canal for three to five minutes. Paracervical blocks can also be performed; however, these may be more painful than the procedure itself.

Other satisfactory endometrial evaluation methods include:

- Curity Isaacs Endometrial Cell Sampler
- The Vabra Aspirator
- The Milex Endometrial Cannula
- Randall or Novak Suction biopsy

Summary

Endometrial biopsies are desirable before beginning estrogen replacement therapy but may only be necessary for those who respond to the progestogen challenge test by bleeding (see Section #9).

Progestogen challenge tests were not performed in the Wilford Hall USAF Medical Center studies (Ref 55, 61). Consequently, most of the endometrial cancers in the estrogen-progestogen users were probably already present from the unopposed estrogens before the progestogen was added. If the progestogen challenge test is utilized as directed, patients with a negative response to the test (no withdrawal bleeding) do not need an endometrial biopsy.

In addition, it is easier to perform the biopsy if the patient returns on the first or second day of withdrawal bleeding. In approximately 10 to 15 percent of postmenopausal women, the cervix is so stenotic that endometrial biopsies are difficult to perform in the office; and withdrawal bleeding dilates the cervix slightly, which facilitates sounding and performing the biopsy in the clinic.

NOTES

#11 Osteoporosis Detection Methods

Types of Methods Available

There are at least four methods of screening women to determine bone loss. These include:

- Regular x-rays
- Single and dual x-ray absorptiometry
- Quantitative computed axial tomography (CAT) scan
- Dual energy x-ray absorptiometry (DEXA)

Regular X-Rays

Regular x-rays of the bones can reveal osteoporosis. However, before osteoporosis can be detected on regular x-rays, a loss of 30 to 40 percent of total bone mass must have occurred. This is a fairly late stage of the disease.

Newer and better methods reveal lesser amounts of bone loss to allow earlier detection and prompt treatment of the condition.

Single and Dual X-Ray Absorptiometry

Photon absorptiometry was developed in the early 1960s while researchers were looking for a method to determine the effect of gravity on bones (particularly, the effect on astronauts). This technique detects small 11. amounts of bone loss, allowing early diagnosis and treatment of osteoporosis. Another advantage is the method's very low radiation exposure, about 1/100 that of standard x-rays.

Single photon absorptiometry is used to measure bone mass in the radius using radioactive iodine (I-131). The amount of radiation that passes through the bone is measured by a detector positioned above the arm, thus determining the thickness of the bone.

Dual photon absorptiometry (DPA) uses radioactive gadolinium (Gd-153) as the radiation source. The DPA has been substituted by the dual energy x-ray densitometry (DEXA) that, instead of using a radioactive source of energy, uses an x-ray beam. It measures bone thickness in the vertebrae (AP or lateral), hip, or femur. Total body calcium can also be measured with this technique. The latest improvement in this method is its detection of bone density of the total body or any part of it, such as:

- Cervical area
- Thoracic or lumbar spine
- Arms
- Legs
- Pelvis
- Ribs

Computers are used with these methods to aid in determining the percent of bone present compared to standards (young-normals) and bone densities found in patients matched for age, sex, and height. The results are plotted on a graph, with the patient's bone thickness or bone mineral density (BMD) on the Y axis and age on the X axis. Standard deviations (SD) are provided for an accurate mode of diagnosis and are represented as every line under the normal mean.

The results are given as a percentage of normal, young women and percentage of age-matched. The standards of bone mass that should be present were worked out at the Mayo Clinic and the University of Wisconsin.

The computer-generated and printed report provides the physician with information about bone mass, including:

- The patient's BMD
- How the BMD compares to others of her age (age-matched), weight, and ethnic background
- How much bone mass has been lost since menopause

The report also indicates on a graph whether the degree of the patient's risk for fracture is:

- Normal
- Mild
- Moderate
- Severe

Quantitative Computed Axial Tomography

A CAT scan was the most accurate measurement of bone until x-ray densitometry was developed. The CAT scan is more expensive; and since it uses x-rays as the radiation source, the amount of radiation exposure is considerably higher than that of dual radiation absorptiometry (13 to 20 times higher).

In young women whose ovaries have been removed, a CAT scan can detect bone loss in the spine very early, as soon as two to four months after surgery (Ref 43). The method is, therefore, very useful in research on osteoporosis, but it is not necessary in evaluating patients for estrogen therapy.

Need for Bone Measurements

Most women do not need any of these osteoporosis screening methods. But for medical researchers, these tests are essential to determine:

- Dosages of estrogen
- The need for supplemental calcium
- Additions of other therapies, e.g.,:
    - Vitamin D
    - Progestogens
    - Diphosphonates

These tests may also be useful in following patients who already have osteoporosis to ensure that its progression has been stopped with the present therapy.

If patients will seek medical evaluation for estrogen deficiency and physicians will treat patients for estrogen deficiency, osteoporosis can be prevented.

It is known that oral therapy with 0.625 mg of conjugated estrogens will prevent osteoporosis in more than 90 percent of postmenopausal women. Active clinical research is being conducted on other types of estrogens to determine the dosages necessary to prevent osteoporosis. Now that 0.5 mg of micronized estradiol is available and 0.625 mg of estropipate is being promoted by different pharmaceutical companies, concern must be expressed that these lower dosages of estrogen are not preventive for the majority of postmenopausal women over the long term (see Section #5).

Biochemical Bone Markers

The new urinary biochemical bone markers, pyridinium crosslinks and telopeptides, may be helpful in monitoring bone loss in estrogen users. Bone markers are not predictive of bone loss in untreated postmenopausal women, nor can they be used to diagnose osteoporosis (Ref 39, 129). Up to 10 percent of postmenopausal estrogen users may be losing bone in spite of adequate estrogen replacement. Where urinary bone markers may be useful is in monitoring estrogen users to be sure their bone mineral density is being maintained. When these bone markers are elevated, which may indicate higher bone loss than replacement, bone density studies should be done to assess the bone adequately.

Until the recent advances in alternative therapies for osteoporosis, e.g., the bisphosphonates and nasal calcitonin (see Sections #5 and #29), little could be done for women losing bone in spite of adequate estrogen therapy. Increasing the estrogen and calcium dosages were of little benefit. Monitoring all estrogen users with bone density studies was very costly and, since little could be done anyway, the cost-to-benefit ratio was out of balance. Now, with the new urinary bone markers, estrogen users can be screened to determine the need for bone density studies so that bisphosphonates or calcitonin can be added to the hormone replacement regimen.

However, estrogen therapy remains the very best prevention and treatment of osteoporosis because of the other benefits of decreasing risks of heart disease, delaying onset of Alzheimer's disease, and reducing colon cancer (see Section #12).

Osteoporosis Screening Clinics

A number of osteoporosis screening clinics are springing up across the U.S. These are beneficial because they are increasing public awareness of osteoporosis.

BMD may be lost due to causes other than estrogen deficiency (e.g., thyroid or parathyroid abnormalities), long-term prednisone therapy, or endocrinopathies in which cortisol is increased. Patients who have undergone gastrointestinal surgeries (e.g., ileostomies, which remove the area where calcium absorption takes place) or who have kidney function impairment (which nullifies vitamin D_3 activity, 1.25 DHC) are subject to bone loss also.

Most women do not need to be screened for osteoporosis and only need to be treated with estrogens if they are estrogen-deficient. However, more than just screening techniques (x-ray densitometry) should be used to follow hormonal response in patients with bone loss.

Although screening is not seen as cost-effective initially, it is in the long-term since osteoporosis is a major public health problem affecting more than 25 million Americans (Ref 120) at an annual cost of $10 to 12 billion. For this reason, prevention is the best way to avoid osteoporosis. It is far better to prevent bone loss than it is to treat osteoporosis.

Who Should Be Screened?

There are certain known factors that increase the risk for osteoporosis (Ref 95). It is not unreasonable to screen women who have multiple risk factors, including:

- White or Asian heritage
- A positive family history of osteoporosis
- Low calcium intake (lifelong)
- Early menopause
- Ovaries removed at a young age
- Sedentary lifestyle
- No children
- Alcohol abuse
- High salt intake
- Cigarette smoking
- High caffeine intake
- High protein intake
- High phosphate intake
- Diseases such as hyperthyroidism
- Certain drugs, e.g., such as steroids

#12 Laboratory and Tests for Early Cancer Detection

Basic Tests

There are a number of basic tests that should be performed when evaluating patients for estrogen replacement therapy. These include:

- Blood pressure
- Electrolytes
- Liver function
- Renal function
- Enzymes
- Complete blood count (CBC)
- Blood indices
- Platelet count
- Thyroxine
- Urinalysis

Additional tests should be obtained if indicated from the history. For example, with a history of nontraumatic thromboembolic disease, the following should be added to the platelet count:

- Prothrombin time
- Partial thromboplastin time
- Antithrombin III

Consideration should be given to fractionalization of cholesterol into HDL and LDL, since LDL cholesterol may be increased after menopause. However, if total cholesterol is below 200 mg/dL and triglycerides are below 150 mg/dL, it is not necessary to fractionate cholesterol levels into HDL and LDL.

These routine tests should be repeated after six months of estrogen therapy and repeated approximately every one to two years thereafter during estrogen therapy.

Follow-up Tests

Annual tests that should be performed include:

- Pap smear in patients with uteri
- Bimanual examination
- Rectal examination

Semiannual tests that should be performed include:

- Blood pressure
- Hemoglobin
- Breast examination

Mammography

Any abnormality of the breasts requires prompt evaluation by mammography and/or direct biopsy. Likewise, any changes in mammary tissue require immediate evaluation. Breast self-examination should be taught to patients and recommended monthly. Semiannual breast exams should be done by the physician, more often if palpable abnormalities are present.

The American Cancer Society's guidelines on mammography should be followed. For the normally palpable breast, mammograms should be performed as follows:

- A baseline mammogram should be obtained at age 40
- Mammogram should be obtained annually after age 40

A controversy has arisen over the cost-effectiveness of mammography screening in women ages 40 to 50 at the U.S. Department of Health and Human Services (Ref 59). However, the American Cancer Society, the American College of Radiology, and ACOG still recommend it; and it has been invaluable in the author's practice.

Estrogen therapy does not increase the risk for breast cancer (see Section #21), but postmenopausal women are reaching the age at which the incidence of breast cancer continuously increases.

Tests for Colon and Rectal Cancer

Colon and rectal cancers are the second most frequent cancers in women (11 percent of all female cancers) and the third leading killer from cancer in women (10 percent of all female cancer deaths). The American Cancer Society estimates that there will be 64,800 new cases of colon and rectal cancers in females in the U.S. during 1997 and that 27,900 women will die from these malignancies this year (Ref 119).

The American Cancer Society recommendations for early detection of colon and rectal cancers include:

- Digital rectal examination annually at age 40
- Stool guaiac slide test annually at age 50
- Sigmoidoscopy every three to five years at age 50

Reduction in Colon Cancer

The most recent benefit shown for hormone replacement therapy is the 30- to 40-percent reduction in colon cancer. Sex steroid hormones modify hepatic cholesterol production and alter bile acid concentration. Increased concentrations of bile acids have long been thought to be important in human colon cancer carcinogenesis. In animal studies, bile acids promote tumors. It has been suggested that exogenous estrogens and progestogen may reduce the secretion of bile acids (Ref 104).

Studies are now confirming that hormone replacement therapy, either estrogens alone or in combination with progestogen, significantly reduces the risk of colon cancer (RR=0.54; 95 percent CI, 0.36

to 0.81) (Ref 112). Overall, postmenopausal hormone use was associated with a 30-percent reduction in colon cancer for ever-use and a 46-percent reduction for recent use.

In a recently published study of 422,373 postmenopausal women, the risk of colon cancer in estrogen users was reduced to RR=0.71 (95 percent CI, 0.61 to 0.83) (Ref 160). With 11 or more years of estrogen use, the reduction was RR=0.54 (95 percent CI, 0.39 to 0.76).

Diagnosis

The diagnosis of menopause can usually be made by history and physical examination, including vaginal hormonal cytology and the progestogen challenge test. If still uncertain, the best single laboratory test is serum FSH.

Postmenopausally, serum FSH and LH values are markedly elevated, with FSH in the range of 75 to 200 mIU/mL and LH in the range of 60 to 90 mIU/mL. Within a year after menses ceases, serum FSH may increase as much as 13-fold, while LH rises approximately threefold. After a further rise in both FSH and LH during early postmenopausal years, there is a gradual decline with age.

Thirty years after menopausal onset, serum gonadotropin levels are only 40 to 50 percent of the maximum reached. However, these levels are still much higher than those found during reproductive years. Serum FSH is more reliable for diagnosis of menopause, since it usually rises more quickly and to higher levels than LH. Also, the midcycle LH surge in ovulating women could be mistaken for a postmenopausal level. If the serum FSH is above 30 mIU/mL, that patient is estrogen-deficient and should be started on replacement therapy.

Serum estrogen levels are unreliable for diagnosis of menopause, since the range of normal is so wide. Serum estradiol varies from five to 25 pg/mL after menopause and from 25 to 75 pg/mL in the follicular phase of reproductive-aged women. Even total urinary estrogens cannot be used, since postmenopausal values are five to 15 micrograms per 24 hours compared to 10 to 25 micrograms per 24 hours during the follicular phase in ovulatory women. Estrogen levels in perimenopausal women should not be used for diagnosis. Peaks and valleys occur in estrogen levels as ovarian function decreases.

NOTES

#13 Oral Estrogens

Clinical Information

When the uterus is present, the patient with menopausal symptoms should be prescribed estrogens and progestogens after proper evaluation (see Section #12) and in the absence of contraindications (see Section #28).

Dosages

Cyclic therapy is usually recommended in order to minimize side effects. However, continuous estrogen therapy is just as safe as long as the estrogen is opposed by a progestogen. Conjugated estrogens at 0.625 mg or equivalent dosages of other natural estrogens (see Table 13.1) can be given according to the calendar from the first through the 25th of the month. The progestogen should be added during the last 13 days of estrogen therapy, from the 13th through the 25th (see Table 16.1). If symptoms recur on the days off estrogens, continuous therapy can be used as long as the estrogen is opposed by a progestogen.

Although lower dosages are available, 0.625 mg of conjugated estrogens is the dosage that has been shown to prevent osteoporosis in more than 90 percent of postmenopausal women. Since prevention of osteoporosis is the major goal of estrogen replacement therapy, this is the lowest dosage that should be used.

If symptoms such as hot flushes persist after two to three months of estrogen therapy, the estrogen dosage can be increased from 0.625 to 0.9 or 1.25 mg of conjugated estrogens. Doses above 1.25 mg are rarely necessary to relieve menopausal symptoms. It is more advisable to add an androgen (see Section #15) than continually to increase the estrogen dose.

Exceptions

There are two exceptions to the normal 0.625 mg estrogen dosage. These are for women who:

- Have had surgical menopause during their reproductive years
- Have osteoporosis

Women with surgical menopause whose ovaries are removed during reproductive years usually require higher dosages of conjugated estrogens (e.g., 1.25 mg) to relieve menopausal symptoms. However, after one to two years, this dose can usually be reduced to 0.625 mg.

Women with osteoporosis also need higher dosages, from 1.25 to 2.5 mg, of conjugated estrogens to reduce fracture rates.

Summary

It is sometimes more difficult to evaluate patients who have had hysterectomies and to initiate proper estrogen therapies for them. If bilateral oophorectomies are also performed during reproductive years, estrogen therapy should be initiated soon afterwards and higher dosages than 1.25 mg conjugated estrogens are often required for prevention of symptoms.

When ovaries are preserved, menopausal symptoms are commonly delayed until the time of natural menopause. However, after a hysterectomy, the ovaries may not continue to function fully until the expected age of natural menopause. Patients presenting with obvious vasomotor symptoms and/or atrophic vaginitis should be started on cyclic estrogen therapy with 0.625 mg of conjugated estrogens from the first through the 25th of each month.

For women who have had hysterectomies and with conservation of ovaries ahd who have minimal symptoms, vaginal hormonal cytology and serum FSH may aid diagnosis. To prevent osteoporosis, estrogen therapy can be instituted when hormonal evidence of menopause exists. In addition, from the 13th through the 25th of each month, cyclic progestogens should be added to the hormone therapy for additional protection of the bones (see Section #5) and the breasts (see Section #21).

TABLE 13.1 – **Oral Estrogens**

NAME	ESTROGEN	MG	MANUFACTURER
Premarin	Conjugated Estrogens	0.3 0.625 0.9 1.25 2.5	Wyeth-Ayerst
Estrace	Micronized Estradiol	0.5 1.0 2.0	Mead Johnson
Estratab	Esterified Estrogens	0.3 0.625 1.25 2.5	Solvay
Ogen	Estropipate	0.625 1.25 2.5 5.0	Abbott Upjohn
Estinyl	Ethinyl Estradiol	0.02 0.05 0.5	Schering
Estrovis	Quinestrol	0.1	Parke-Davis

#14 Non-Oral Estrogens

Estrogen Vaginal Cream

Estrogen vaginal cream is the longest available and probably the most useful of the non-oral estrogens. In creams, estrogens are well-absorbed through the vaginal mucosa so that good systemic levels are obtained as well as the local beneficial effects. Vaginal creams probably provide the quickest response and subsequent relief of symptoms of atrophic vaginitis, such as:

- Vaginal irritation
- Pruritus
- Vaginal dryness
- Dyspareunia

One common course of treatment is to apply Premarin vaginal cream, 1 g daily (see Table 14.1). Usually, oral estrogens are started simultaneously. After two weeks of double therapy, the maintenance dosage of the vaginal cream can often be reduced to three times weekly or can be entirely eliminated.

However, some patients on oral estrogens may continue to require estrogen vaginal cream for maintenance of the vaginal mucosa. Also, some women may not respond adequately to oral estrogens alone, developing dryness or pruritus of the vagina while on therapy. Instead of increasing the oral estrogen dosage, these women frequently benefit more from the addition of estrogen vaginal cream to the therapeutic routine.

Use of oral estrogens has been questioned because of portal absorption and liver metabolism as well as the risk of cholelithiasis. With the first liver-pass, hepatic enzymatic changes may be induced that alter various biochemical parameters (Ref 21). Oral therapy may result in estrogen being delivered directly into hepatic tissue via the portal circulation. This could possibly result in changes in the rates of synthesis of certain hepatically derived proteins and globulins, such as:

- Renin substrate
- Cortisol-binding globulin (CBG)
- Sex hormone-binding globulin (SHBG)
- Antithrombin III

Most of these changes are minor and may not be clinically significant.

Non-oral routes of administration deliver the estrogen directly into the systemic circulation and, thus, may cause less marked changes in hepatic biosynthesis because the portal system is by-passed. However, at least one of the benefits of oral therapy, the increase in HDL cholesterol, may be delayed by non-oral administration. Apparently, the first liver-pass induces this antiatherogenic lipoprotein more quickly.

Saturated Vaginal Rings

Silastic vaginal rings can be saturated with sex steroids, releasing fairly constant amounts of estrogen and/or progestogen into peripheral blood. Whether this method will be widely accepted by patients remains to be determined, but cyclic therapy with the natural steroids (estradiol and progesterone) can be provided through the vaginal mucosa.

An estradiol vaginal ring containing 2 mg of estradiol (Estring; Pharmacia, Upjohn) has just been approved by the FDA for treatment of atrophic vaginitis. There is little to no systemic absorption, so it is intended for local use only. One ring will last for 90 days. There is improvement in vaginal mucosal epithelium after 12 weeks, and the vaginal pH is restored to normal.

In contrast to oral micronized estradiol, vaginal estradiol:

- Provides a low estrone-to-estradiol ratio
- Does not induce a high postmedication estrogen peak
- Reaches the peripheral circulation without passing the enterohepatic circulation

Estradiol Subcutaneous Pellets

Subcutaneous implantation of 17β-estradiol pellets, the principal human estrogen, has been available for more than 50 years until it was temporarily banned by the FDA in 1980 for lack of efficacy and safety studies. These pellets should again become available in 1997. They are available from certain pharmacies.

The main use of estradiol pellets has been by patients who could not use oral estrogens because of a lack of response or because of side effects associated with oral estrogens. Estradiol pellets have been shown to be very effective in relieving menopausal symptoms (Ref 148), including:

- Hot flushes (or flashes)
- Insomnia
- Dyspareunia

Side effects, which occur in five to eight percent of oral estrogen users, are diminished in those who use pellets because of the use of the major ovarian estrogen.

When combined with subcutaneous testosterone pellets, estradiol implants are particularly effective in treating psychosexual problems such as loss of libido and anorgasmia, which may not respond to estrogen alone (Ref 69, 149). Estradiol pellets provide more normal estrone-to-estradiol ratios than oral estrogens and also provide more constant estrogen levels than any parenteral form of estrogen administration.

Transdermal Estradiol

The transdermal system of estrogen replacement therapy is another form of non-oral administration. This system has been shown to be clinically effective in relieving menopausal symptoms. Comparative studies indicate that the transdermal system provides more normal estrone-to-estradiol ratios than oral estrogens.

Estraderm at 0.05 to 0.1 mg daily elicited many of the desirable actions of estrogen while avoiding the pharmacologic effects of oral estrogens on hepatic proteins (Ref 20, 21). The patches are placed on the skin at 8:00 a.m. Monday and 8:00 p.m. Thursday, since estradiol levels are effective for three and one-half days. Patches should be used continuously, since symptoms may return when patches are removed because of rapidly falling estradiol levels.

New transdermal systems have recently become available: Climara and Vivelle. Climara is a weekly patch available in both 0.05 and 0.1 mg per day dosages. Skin irritation seems to be less, although the patch is left on the skin for a longer duration. This patch has no alcohol (acid alcohol is a primary skin irritant).

Vivelle is another new matrix patch with no alcohol for reduced skin irritation. It is available in four dosages: 0.0375, 0.05, 0.075, and 0.1 mg per day.

Although there are few or no undesirable effects with transdermal systems, endometrial proliferation is normal and an oral progesterone must be given for 10 to 13 days. Transdermal estradiol takes longer to produce a rise in HDL cholesterol than do oral estrogens (Ref 143). Over the long-term, patches should be just as protective from atherosclerotic heart disease, especially with the 0.1 mg estradiol dosage.

TABLE14.1 – **Estrogen Vaginal Cream and Ring**

NAME	ESTROGEN	MG/GM	MANUFACTURER
Premarin Vaginal Cream	Conjugated estrogens	0.625 mg	Wyeth-Ayerst
Estrace Vaginal Cream	17β-estradiol	0.1 mg	Mead Johnson
Ogen Vaginal Cream	Estropipate	1.5 mg	Abbott
Ortho Dienestrol Cream	Dienestrol	0.01%	Ortho
Estragard Cream	Dienestrol	0.01%	Solvay
Diethylstilbestrol Suppositories	Diethylstilbestrol	0.1 mg 0.5 mg	Lilly
Estring	Estradiol	2 mg total	Pharmacia, Upjohn

TABLE 14.2 – **Parenteral Estrogens**

NAME	ESTROGEN	MG/ML	MANUFACTURER
Depo-Estradiol	estradiol cypionate	1 mg 5 mg	Upjohn
Delestrogen	estradiol valerate	10 mg 20 mg 40 mg	Squibb
Estraval	estradiol valerate	10 mg 20 mg	Solvay
Estrapel*	estradiol pellet	25 mg pellet	Bartor
Estraderm	transdermal estradiol	0.05 mg/day 0.1 mg/day	Ciba-Geigy
Climara	transdermal estradiol	0.05 mg/day 0.1 mg/day	Berlex
Vivelle	transdermal estradiol	0.0375 mg/day 0.05 mg/day 0.075 mg/day 0.1 mg/day	Ciba-Geneva

*Available from certain pharmacies

#15 Androgens

Clinical Information

Estrogens give relief of most menopausal symptoms. However, it sometimes becomes necessary to add androgens to hormone replacement therapy. Up to 75 percent of estrogen production is lost after menopause, but up to 50 percent of androgen production can also be lost when ovaries cease to function or are surgically removed. If symptoms persist, it is best to add a low dose of androgen to the estrogen replacement regimen than to continue increasing the estrogen dosage beyond 1.25 mg of conjugated estrogens (see Table 15.1).

Potential benefits of androgens include alleviation of:

- Hot flushes (or flashes)
- Lethargy
- Endogenous depression
- Kraurosis vulvae (with use of one- to two-percent testosterone cream)
- Nocturia and incontinence
- Fibrocystic disease of the breast
- Headaches (migrainoid)

Although estrogens will alleviate both hot flushes and genital atrophy, the addition of an androgen will help overcome fatigue. When estrogens are contraindicated (as in patients with breast cancer), androgens alone may be helpful to relieve vasomotor symptoms and improve the psyche. However, they are of little value in treatment of genital atrophy and probably do not prevent osteoporosis in the dosages that can be used.

Some postmenopausal women complain of hirsutism before any hormone replacement. This is probably due to a relative imbalance of endogenous estrogens and androgens where estrogen levels decrease more than testosterone levels. Typically manifested by an increase in upper lip hair or small moustache, this usually lessens after estrogen replacement.

Androgen therapy can aggravate:

- Preexisting hirsutism
- Acne
- Skin oiliness

If there are good results from the androgen but aggravation of hirsutism or acne, reducing the androgen dosage and/or increasing the estrogen dosage may help. Spironolactone at 25 mg four times daily may also be added to the estrogen-androgen combination so that the benefits of the androgen can be continued.

Research

In one study, patients experienced relief of hot flushes with non-oral therapies (Ref 69) as follows:

- Ninety-six percent with estradiol pellets
- Eighty-nine percent with estradiol pellets p testosterone
- Fifty-five percent with testosterone alone
- Sixteen percent with placebo

Estrogen alone gave less benefit than estrogen-androgen pellets, which:

- Increased feelings of well-being
- Improved libido
- Relieved endogenous depression
- Lessened migrainoid headaches

In postmenopausal women, androgens added to estrogen replacement commonly improved problems with:

- Libido
- Sexual response
- Anorgasmia

An increase in libido occurred (Ref 69) in:

- More than 65 percent of those treated with androgens
- 12.3 percent of those receiving estrogens
- Only 1.8 percent of those taking the placebo

In a study in which 76 women received pellet implants of 50 mg estradiol, a combination of 50 mg estradiol and 100 mg testosterone, or placebo every six months, only those on the combination estrogen-androgen experienced a decided increase in sexual response and frequency of coitus (Ref 148, 150). The addition of testosterone implants also increased the frequency and intensity of orgasmic responses.

Recommendations

Available forms of androgen and estrogen-androgen combinations are found in Table 15.1.

ORAL THERAPY

Estratest or Estratest H.S. is a better-balanced combination than Premarin with methyltestosterone. Therapy should be cyclic from the first through the 25th of the month to minimize side effects, and a progestogen should be added from the 13th through the 25th of the month. Although androgens may suppress the endometrium slightly, most patients on estrogen-androgen combinations will have withdrawal menses from the progestogen challenge test.

INJECTABLES

Depo-Testadiol 1 cc IM will usually relieve symptoms for four weeks.

SUBCUTANEOUS PELLETS

Estradiol pellets are available in the U.S. from certain pharmacies. Testosterone pellets are the only form of androgen therapy for females available that use the natural hormone, which reduces potential side effects. A testosterone patch was released in 1994 to treat males; however, this must be applied to the scrotum where the skin is thin enough to absorb enough testosterone, and there is no comparable skin on women for placement.

For women, one or two 75 mg pellets of testosterone may be implanted subcutaneously (these last four to six months) with the estrogen replacement given orally or by transdermal patch (Estraderm). Oral progestogens should also be added from the 13th to the 25th of the month.

TABLE 15.1 – **Androgens**

	NAME	ANDROGEN	MG/ML	MANUFACTURER
Oral Androgens	Oreton	methyltestosterone	5 mg	Schering
	Metandren	methyltestosterone	5 mg	Ciba
	Halotestin	fluoxymesterone	2 mg 5 mg	Upjohn
	Fluoxymesterone	fluoxymesterone	5 mg	Solvay
Injectables	Depo-testosterone	testosterone cypionate	100 mg/ml 200 mg/ml	Upjohn
	Delatestryl	testosterone enanthate	100 mg/ml	Squibb
	Testopel	testosterone pellets	75 mg	Bartor

Estrogen/Androgen Combinations	Estratest tablets	esterified estrogens methyltestosterone	1.25 mg 2.5 mg	Solvay
	Estratest H.S. tablets	esterified estrogens methyltestosterone	0.625 mg 1.25 mg	Solvay
	Premarin with Methyltestosterone	conjugated estrogens methyltestosterone	1.25 mg 10 mg	Wyeth-Ayerst
	Premarin with Methyltestosterone	conjugated estrogens methyltestosterone	0.625 mg 5 mg	Wyeth-Ayerst
	Depo-Testadiol	estradiol cypionate testosterone cypionate	2 mg 50 mg	Upjohn
	Estrapel*	estradiol pellet (given with testosterone pellets)	25 mg	Various pharmacies

*Available from certain pharmacies.

#16 Progestogens

Clinical Information

There are three ways that progestogens are commonly used in estrogen replacement therapy. These are:

- Annually, in the progestogen challenge test
- Cyclically, to oppose estrogen effects
- Continuously, to oppose estrogen and induce amenorrhea

Progestogen Challenge Test

The progestogen challenge test should be performed on all climacteric women who have intact uteri and who are:

- Asymptomatic and having regular annual examination
- Symptomatic and are being evaluated for estrogen therapy
- Currently on unopposed estrogen therapy

In the testing procedure, the patient takes 13 days of progestogen (see Table 16.1). If withdrawal bleeding occurs, progestogens should be added to the estrogen therapy from the 13th to the 25th of each monthly cycle. If there is no response, the progestogen challenge test should be repeated annually for asymptomatic women not using hormones.

Cyclic Use of Progestogens

Progestogens are increasingly being added to estrogen replacement therapy for postmenopausal women. In the 1970s, studies revealed that unopposed estrogen replacement therapy increases the risk of endometrial cancer. Therefore, reasons for adding progestogens to estrogen replacement include:

- Prevention of endometrial cancer
- Reduction in risk of breast cancer
- Promotion of new bone formation
- Prevention and treatment of osteoporosis

Some troublesome effects of unopposed estrogen (e.g., breast tenderness) may be alleviated by adding progestogens. Although added progestogen may aggravate mastodynia when initiating therapy, this usually abates with time. Edema, bloating, and irritability are more frequent in women taking unopposed estrogens but are sometimes aggravated by added progestogen.

Other uses of progestogens during the climacteric include:

- Preventing vasomotor flushes
- Avoiding annual endometrial biopsies
- Decreasing the frequency of D&Cs performed for abnormal postmenopausal bleeding

One major drawback is that the same contraindications are listed for progestogens as for estrogens. However, this labeling should not preclude physicians from using their best judgment in the interest of their patients.

There is no good evidence that progestogens have an adverse reaction on coagulation factors or mammary tissue in humans.

There are also concerns about the long-term effects of progestogens, particularly with possible adverse effects on HDL cholesterol (see Section #26). Some patients are reluctant to resume menstruation and sometimes experience premenstrual-like symptoms during progestogen therapy. However, after menopause, menstrual effects are lessened for patients taking progestogens, including:

- Reduced menstrual flow (three to four days)
- Lessened dysmenorrhea
- Lessened PMS

Research has demonstrated a reduction in abnormal postmenopausal bleeding. In one study, abnormal bleeding occurred in 23.3 percent of nonusers of hormones, 14.2 percent of users of estrogen alone, and in only 3.9 percent of estrogen-progestogen users (Ref 60).

Although any unscheduled bleeding should be promptly investigated, annual endometrial biopsies are not required for users of progestogens. One study showed that hyperplasia or neoplasia occurred in 8.1 percent of nonusers, 7.9 percent of estrogen users, and 0.9 percent of estrogen-progestogen users.

Adding Progestogen to Estrogen Replacement

Patients receiving oral estrogens from the first through the 25th of each month should have the progestogen added (see Table 16.1) from the 13th through the 25th for the benefit of the bones and the breasts (see Sections #5 and #21). This includes women who have had hysterectomies.

Women on continuous estrogen, injectables, or estradiol pellet implants may be given the progestogen the first 13 days of each month.

For initial therapy, C-21 progestogens (e.g., Provera 10 mg) should be chosen for women with histories of breast problems such as fibrocystic disease or mastodynia. The 19-nor-steroid progestogens (e.g., Aygestin 2.5 or 5 mg) are best for those with histories of heavy or prolonged menstrual periods.

Studies show that less than 10 mg of Provera may not be protective for the endometrium (Ref 50). Although 5 mg of Aygestin is the recommended starting dosage, as little as 1 mg of norethindrone may be protective for the endometrium. Therefore, the trend is toward lower dosage of the 19-nor-steroid progestogens (e.g., 2.5 mg of Aygestin).

Injectable progestogens are not recommended for postmenopausal women with intact uteri, since the duration of action is irregular and breakthrough bleeding may result.

The continuous combined, low dosage estrogen-progestogen therapy is not recommended because of increasing reports of endometrial cancer on this regimen (see Section #20). The cyclic combined regimen with Premarin (0.625 to 0.9 mg) and Provera (2.5 mg) is preferred from the first through the 25th of each month. This produces more amenorrhea (75 percent) than the continuous combined method (60 to 65 percent); and when bleeding does occur, it is only one or two days of spotting on the 26th or 27th of the month. It should be more endometrial-protective since it is important to interrupt the progestogen for a few days each month to allow any build-up of endometrium to be shed.

Side Effects of Estrogen-Progestogen Therapy

The major side effect of estrogen-progestogen therapy is that 97 percent of patients have withdrawal bleeding until age 60, with 60 percent of patients continuing withdrawal bleeding after age 65. In addition, five to 10 percent of patients experience:

- Breast tenderness
- Edema
- Bloating
- Premenstrual irritability
- Lower abdominal cramps
- Dysmenorrhea

Patient acceptance of withdrawal bleeding has been good once the benefits are clearly explained. However, patients do not have to accept continued menses with alternative methods of combination estrogen-progestogen therapy.

Side effects may be managed by:

- Decreasing the estrogen dosage
- Adding a mild diuretic:
  - HCTZ, 25 to 50 mg, OR
  - Spironolactone, 25 to 50 mg
- Changing to another progestogen

For patients who cannot tolerate any oral progestogen, progesterone suppositories (50 mg daily) may be used in divided dosages (Ref 56). Also, oral micronized progesterone is available from certain pharmacies and should be commercially available. The dosage is 300 mg daily in divided dosages, 100 mg in the morning and 200 mg at bedtime, since the major side effect is drowsiness.

General aches and pains can be dealt with by using a prostaglandin-inhibiting analgesic such as:

- Aspirin
- Motrin, 400 to 800 mg four times daily
- Ibuprofen; Pharmacia, Upjohn
- Naproxen, 250 to 500 mg three times daily
- Naprosyn; Syntex
- Anaprox, 275 to 550 mg three times daily (Naproxen Sodium, Syntex)
- Ponstel, 250 mg four times daily (mefenamic acid; Parke-Davis)

TABLE16.1 –**Progestogens**

NAME	PROGESTOGEN	MG	MANUFACTURER
Provera	medroxyprogesterone acetate	2.5, 5, 10	Pharmacia,Upjohn
Curretab	medroxyprogesterone acetate	10	Solvay
Cyrin	medroxyprogesterone acetate	10	Lederle
Amen	medroxyprogesterone acetate	10	Carnrick
Aygestin	norethindrone acetate	5	Lederle
Megace	megestrol acetate	20, 40	Bristol-Myers
Ovrette	norgestrel	0.075	Wyeth-Ayerst
Micronor	norethindrone	0.35	Ortho
Nor-Q.D.	norethindrone	0.35	Syntex
	progesterone vaginal suppositories	25, 50	–
	oral micronized progesterone	50, 100	–

#17 Oral Contraceptives

There are greater doses of estrogen and progestogen in oral contraceptives than are needed to treat postmenopausal women. Even the lowest dose oral contraceptive has 20 µg of ethinyl estradiol and 1 mg of norethindrone acetate. Five µg of ethinyl estradiol, particularly when combined with a progestogen, will prevent osteoporosis and relieve menopausal symptoms. However, with the increasing recognition of side benefits, rather than side effects, birth control pills should be encouraged for perimenopausal nonsmokers needing family planning. Smokers ages 40 and older should be encouraged to stop smoking so that they can also reap these benefits.

Noncontraceptive Health Benefits

Noncontraceptive health benefits of oral contraceptives are:

- Decreased risks of:
  - Endometrial cancer
  - Ovarian cancer
  - Ovarian cysts
- Less benign breast disease
- Probably less breast cancer
- Treatment of:
  - Dysfunctional uterine bleeding
  - Dysmenorrhea
  - Hirsutism
  - Acne
  - Endometriosis
- Decreased:
  - Iron deficiency anemia
  - Thyroid disease
- Less rheumatic arthritis
- Effective contraception

- Decreased:
  - Ectopic pregnancy
  - Pelvic inflammatory disease
- Increased bone mass

Breast Cancer

Although this remains controversial, there is no evidence from the more than 100 studies that oral contraceptive use increases the risk of carcinoma of the breast (Ref 134). In fact, the contrary could be true. In one of the largest studies of women whose carcinoma of the breast was diagnosed between ages 45 and 54, those who had used birth control pills had a slightly decreased risk of breast cancer (RR=0.9; 95 percent CI, 0.8 to 1.0) (Ref 163). Among these women, the risk estimates decreased significantly ($P \leq 0.01$) with increasing time between first and last use.

Not only do oral contraceptives significantly reduce the risk of benign breast disease, but birth control pills and progestogens reverse both intraductal hyperplasia and atypia of the breast, which may be precancerous lesions (Ref 157).

#18 Calcium Supplements

Clinical Information

Bone loss due to osteoporosis is associated with alterations in calcium metabolism yielding negative calcium balance. Although calcium intake does not decrease at the time of menopause and calcium absorption does not vary greatly, a rise in fasting urinary calcium is found at about this time (Ref 47).

As determined by the NIH Consensus Conference on Osteoporosis, the American diet is deficient in calcium intake, particularly among women who diet to maintain a thin figure (Ref 120). The usual daily intake of elemental calcium in the U.S., 450 to 550 mg, is below the National Research Council's recommended dietary allowance (RDA) of 800 mg per day. Calcium metabolic balance studies indicate a daily requirement of 1,000 mg of elemental calcium for premenopausal and estrogen-treated postmenopausal women. Postmenopausal women who are not treated with estrogens require 1,500 mg or more daily for calcium balance.

Calcium Level Changes

Changes in urinary calcium levels are difficult to detect since 24-hour collections reflect absorbed dietary calcium. Patients must be studied in a fasting state when urinary calcium derives primarily from bone.

By comparing fasting calcium levels in hysterectomized women who also had bilateral oophorectomy to those who had ovarian conservation, the increase in resorption of calcium from bone can be related to reduced ovarian estrogens (Ref 47). Both fasting plasma and urinary hydroxyproline confirm that the increased calcium excretion is due to increased bone resorption of calcium. Women undergoing natural menopause have similar changes in calcium metabolism. Postmenopausal women show a higher morning fasting urinary calcium-to-creatinine ratio than premenopausal women.

The increase in fasting serum or urinary calcium that follows either natural menopause or bilateral oophorectomy is reversible with estrogen therapy. Estrogen administration also stimulates calcitonin production, which is decreased after menopause, and may affect bone calcium indirectly since calcitonin is known to inhibit bone resorption. Adding progestogen to estrogen replacement therapy enhances the effects of the estrogen, thereby promoting new bone formation (Ref 154).

Recommendations

As recommended by the NIH Consensus Conference on Osteoporosis, calcium supplements are essential but of secondary importance to estrogen replacement. Weight-bearing exercise was the third recommendation. A few studies have shown a reduction in fracture rate with calcium alone. However, most studies have also used estrogen replacement plus calcium.

Calcium carbonate is the most widely-studied calcium and probably the best absorbed, with 40 percent absorbed as elemental calcium. Other calcium products can be used, but amounts absorbed as elemental calcium vary. For example, only 10 percent of calcium lactate is absorbed as calcium. Most of the calcium makers now list the amount of elemental calcium in their products rather than the total mg of calcium in each tablet (see Table 18.1).

Calcium supplementation should be started by age 35 to 40 since this is when women have peak bone mass. Women whose diets are markedly deficient in calcium should start supplementation earlier (Ref 120). The more bone mass a women has entering menopause, the more she is apt to retain.

The major sources of calcium in the U.S. diet are milk and dairy products. Each eight ounce glass of milk contains 275 to 300 mg of calcium. Skim milk may actually contain more calcium. Other dietary sources of calcium include:

- Low fat yogurt
- Cheese
- Fish, particularly those canned with bones
- Clams, oysters, and shrimp
- Spinach, broccoli, leafy vegetables
- Peanuts, almonds, brazil nuts
- Tofu
- Calcium-fortified orange juice

Other agents that may be helpful in preventing osteoporosis include (Ref 98):

- Vitamin D or analogues
- Sodium fluoride
- Calcitriol
- Calcitonin
- Anabolic steroids
- Thiazide diuretics
- Magnesium
- Etidronate
- Alendronate

More research needs to be done with these agents before they can be widely recommended. Calcitonin (Calcimar, USV Laboratories) at 100 IU daily by injection (subcutaneous or IM) is probably the best substitute for estrogen replacement when estrogens are contraindicated.

Intranasal calcitonin (Miacalcin by Sandoz) has recently been approved for use in the U.S. An intranasal daily dose of 200 IU was able to maintain bone mass in both the spine and femur (Ref 66, 124). Calcitonin seems to be more effective in the period more than five years after menopause but not as effective as estrogen and the bisphosphonates.

TABLE 18.1 – **Calcium Supplements**

NAME	CALCIUM	ELEMENTAL CA	MANUFACTURER
Os-Cal 500	calcium carbonate	500 mg	Marion
Os-Cal 250	calcium carbonate + Vit D	250 mg	Marion
Posture	calcium phosphate	600 mg	Whitehall
Posture with D	calcium phosphate + Vit D	600 mg	Whitehall
Caltrate 600	calcium carbonate	600 mg	Lederle
Caltrate 600 + Vit D	calcium carbonate + Vit D	600 mg	Lederle
Citracal	calcium citrate	200 mg	Mission
Calcet	calcium lactate	152.8 mg	Mission
	calcium gluconate		
	calcium carbonate		
Nutravescent	calcium citrate + V + D	500 mg	Northhampton
Tums	calcium carbonate	200 mg	Smithkline Beecham
Tums Ex	calcium carbonate	300 mg	
Tums 500	calcium carbonate	500 mg	

NOTES

#19 Endometrial Hyperplasia

Research

Hyperplasia of the endometrium has been established as a precancerous lesion in some women. In a prospective study of 562 women with adenomatous hyperplasia, 18.5 percent developed cancer after a few years. By the tenth year, the incidence of adenocarcinoma rose to 30 percent (Ref 71).

In another study, 115 patients with hyperplasia or adenocarcinoma *in situ* were followed for two to eight years without any therapy, either hysterectomy or hormonal manipulation. A significant number developed invasive adenocarcinoma (Ref 158), including:

- 26.7 percent of those with adenomatous hyperplasia
- 81.8 percent of those with atypical hyperplasia
- 100 percent of those with adenocarcinoma *in situ*

Of the 31 patients with endometrial cancer in the Wilford Hall USAF Medical Center study, 11 (39.3 percent) had a previous diagnosis of hyperplasia from four months to eight years before detection of cancer (Ref 53). Although earlier studies contend that adenomatous hyperplasia may be precancerous, any degree of hyperplasia may be significant since six of these 11 patients had only benign or cystic hyperplasia, yet developed endometrial cancer in a relatively short period of time.

In a five-year prospective study, 325 women were found to have varying degrees of endometrial hyperplasia (Ref 53). They were treated with progestogens for seven to 10 days each month for three to six months and curettage was repeated after therapy. Hyperplasia reversed to normal endometrium in 307 (94.5 percent). Of the 18 patients with persistent hyperplasia, 14 had been given progestogens for only seven days each month, and only four patients with persistent hyperplasia had been treated for 10 days monthly (see Table 19.1).

For the past 10 years at the Medical College of Georgia, every endometrial hyperplasia has been successfully reversed to a normal endometrium within six months by using progestogens 13 days monthly (see Table 19.2).

Hyperplasia and Estrogen Replacement Therapy

Unopposed estrogens have a role in the development of endometrial hyperplasia and neoplasia, primarily because of incomplete shedding of the endometrium. Progesterone or progestogen therapy ensures more complete sloughing of the endometrium, leaving behind fewer glands and cells for continued proliferation and growth. The protective action of progestogens on the endometrium is primarily physical. However, additional actions of both natural progesterone and synthetic progestogens may be important. Progestogens decrease estrogen receptors in endometrial cells and induce estradiol dehydrogenase and isocitrate activity, which are the mechanisms by whose means these cells metabolize estrogens.

Recommendations for Treatment

The preferred method of treatment of endometrial hyperplasia is an initial curettage followed by a course of progestogen therapy (see Table 16.1). Aygestin 5 mg or Provera 10 mg should be taken for 13 days monthly. After six months of progestogen therapy, the curettage should be repeated. If the endometrial hyperplasia is persistent, hysterectomy is recommended.

If the patient is on estrogen therapy, discontinuance is not necessary during the six months of progestogen therapy. The hyperplasia will reverse equally well on combined estrogen-progestogen therapy.

TABLE 19.1 – **Effects of Progestogens on Endometrial Hyperplasia**
Total Numbers of Patients: 325

PATHOLOGY BEFORE THERAPY	NO. OF PATIENTS
Benign hyperplasia	196
Cystic hyperplasia	34
Adenomatous hyperplasia	28
Atypical adenomatous hyperplasia	67
ENDOMETRIUM AFTER THERAPY	**NO. OF PATIENTS**
Proliferative	156
Secretory	69
Atrophic	53
Dyssynchronous maturation	29
Benign hyperplasia	12
Adenomatous hyperplasia	4
Atypical adenomatous hyperplasia	2

TABLE 19.2 – **Reversal of Hyperplasia with Increased Duration of Progestogens**

Number of Patients with Hyperplasia	Duration of Progestogens (Days)	Persistent Hyperplasia	% Reversal
72	7	14	80.6
253	10	4	98.4
45	13	0	100.0

NOTES

#20 Endometrial Cancer

Clinical Information

Unopposed estrogen therapy increases the risk of endometrial cancer, although the magnitude has been exaggerated by the methodology used in retrospective studies (Ref 99, 137, 140, 166). Progestogen added to estrogen replacement therapy for 12 to 14 days per month reduces the risk of endometrial adenocarcinoma to less than that of untreated women (Ref 50, 52, 53, 55, 58, 73, 115, 153). For those not needing estrogen replacement, use of the progestogen challenge test to screen asymptomatic postmenopausal women can reduce adenocarcinoma of the endometrium (Ref 50, 55, 58).

Not all postmenopausal women need estrogen. Many produce sufficient endogenous estrogens to remain asymptomatic and prevent the metabolic changes of long-term estrogen deficiency in later life. However, within this group may be those in need of progestogen to prevent endometrial hyperplasia, possibly leading to endometrial carcinoma. The progestogen challenge test (see Section #9) was devised to identify those in this high-risk group. A positive response to this test (withdrawal bleeding) indicates that 13 days per month of progestogen therapy should be continued for as long as withdrawal bleeding occurs in order to ensure complete endometrial shedding.

Research

During the five years of prospective study and four years of follow-up at Wilford Hall USAF Medical Center from 1975 to 1983 (Figure 20.1), 5,563 post-menopausal women were registered in the hormone user survey (Ref 53). However, approximately

40 percent had hysterectomies and consequently were not at risk for endometrial cancer. Adenocarcinoma of the endometrium was diagnosed in 31 patients during 27,243 patient-years of observation, for an overall incidence of 113.8 per 100,000 women per year (see Table 20.1).

The largest group of patients, the estrogen-progestogen users with 16,327 patient-years of observation, was found to have eight cancers for an annual incidence of 49.0 per 100,000 women. The highest incidence of endometrial carcinoma was observed in the unopposed estrogen users, in whom 10 cancers were detected during 2,560 patient-years, for an incidence of 390.6 per 100,000 women. The second highest incidence was 11 cancers in the nonusers of hormones during 4,480 patient-years of observation, for an incidence of 245.5 per 100,000 women. Only two endometrial cancers were observed in the estrogen vaginal cream users, and no malignancies occurred in either the progestogen or androgen users. This group consisted primarily of progestogen users, women who had been identified as being at increased risk for adenocarcinoma by the progestogen challenge test and who were being treated with cyclic progestogens only.

Other studies have demonstrated the efficacy of progestogens in protecting estrogen users from adenocarcinoma. One reported no endometrial cancers in 72 estrogen-progestogen users, but 11 cancers in 207 patients treated with unopposed estrogens (Ref 73). In a double-blind study, no adenocarcinomas were diagnosed in the 84 patients using estrogen-progestogen for 10 years, but one endometrial cancer occurred in the 84 placebo users (Ref 108). Studies from England have not uncovered any increased risk for endometrial malignancy in estrogen-treated postmenopausal women, because they routinely add a progestogen (Ref 153). However, a 15-percent endometrial hyperplasia rate was observed in the unopposed estrogen users before progestogens were added (Ref 153).

The increasing addition of progestogens to estrogen replacement therapy is already having a beneficial effect on the national incidence of endometrial cancer. Figure 20.2 compares the 1973 to 1977 SEER incidence of endometrial cancer by age when mostly unopposed estrogen was used (Ref 111) to the 1981 to 1985 SEER incidence when progestogens were being increasingly added to estrogen replacement (Ref 4). The trend shown is a shift downward in incidence and to a later age, confirming the effectiveness of adding progestogens.

Cases of Endometrial Cancer with Estrogen-Progestogen Use

In a current review, there were 66 cases of endometrial cancer reported with estrogen-progestogen use (Ref 58). The vast majority occurred when too low a dosage of progestogen or too short a duration of progestogen was given. There are no cases of endometrial cancer reported when 10 mg of medroxyprogesterone acetate or 5 mg of norethindrone acetate was prescribed for 12 to 14 days each month.

The continuous combined method of hormone replacement may not be fully endometrial-protective, since 15 of the reported cases of cancer were using this regimen (Ref 26, 37, 63, 67, 92). In addition to these 15 reported cases, the author has learned of 56 additional cases of endometrial cancer, including two deaths, for a total of 71; this may only be the tip of the iceberg. Since these cases did not begin to appear until a decade of ever increasing usage of the continuous combined hormone replacement regimen and most occurred after two to four years of amenorrhea, the one to three years' published studies were of insufficient duration to demonstrate safety. It may be very important to withdraw the progestogen for a few days each month to allow any build-up of endometrium to be shed. This is the way that the normal ovulatory cycle, sequential estrogen-progestogen therapy, and oral contraceptives work to decrease the risk of endometrial cancer.

A Better Method?

For the past seven years, the author has used the cyclic combined regimen to produce amenorrhea (Ref 33). Low dosage estrogen and progestogen (2.5 mg of medroxyprogesterone acetate or 2.5 mg of norethindrone acetate) are given by the calendar from the first through the 25th of each month.

This is clinically superior to the continuous combined method in that after comparable spotting during the first month of therapy, there is less breakthrough bleeding, usually one or two days of spotting on the 26th or 27th. More women will become amenorrheic by four months (75 percent) compared to 60 to 65 percent with the continuous combined regimen.

When bleeding does occur with the cyclic combined method, it is usually only one or two days of spotting on the 26th or 27th, which most women can accept when full explanation and reassurance are given.

Whether the cyclic combined regimen will be more endometrial-protective than the continuous combined method remains to be proven, since there is only seven years of experience. Theoretically, the regimen should be protective, since discontinuing the progestogen should allow for shedding any build-up of endometrium.

TABLE 20.1 – **Incidence of Endometrial Cancer at Wilford Hall USAF Medical Center: 1975-1983**

THERAPY GROUP	PATIENT-YEARS OF OBSERVATION	PATIENTS WITH CANCER	INCIDENCE (PER 100,000)
Estrogen-Progestogen Users	16,327	8	49.0
Unopposed Estrogen Users	2,560	10	390.6
Estrogen Vaginal Cream Users	2,716	2	73.6
Progestogen Users	1,160	0	×
Non-Users	4,480	11	245.5
TOTAL	27,243	31	113.8

FIGURE 20.1—**Incidence of Endometrial Cancer**

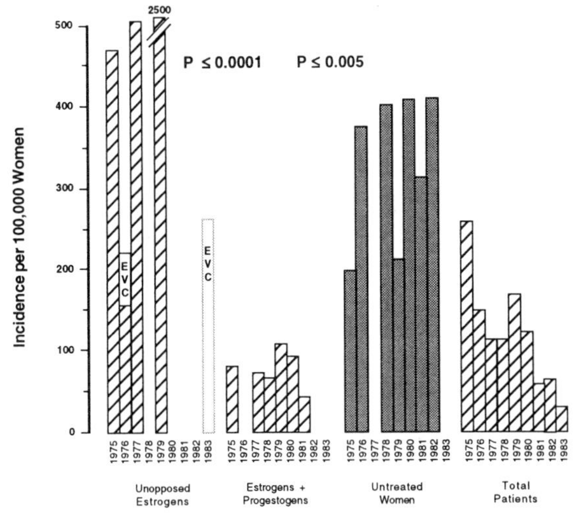

Incidence of endometrial cancer in the various treatment groups compared with untreated from 1975-1983 (Reproduced with permission from Gambrell) (Ref 53).

FIGURE 20.2—**Changing Incidence of Endometrial Cancer**

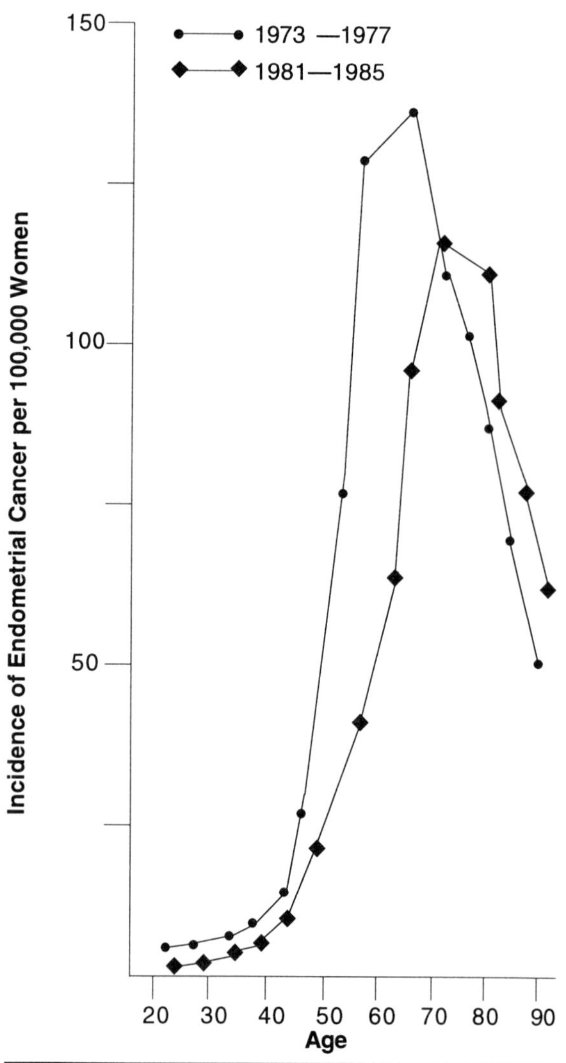

FIGURE 20.2—The shifting of endometrial cancer in women by age between 1973-1977 and 1981-1985.

NOTES

#21 Breast Cancer

Clinical Information

Breast cancer is the most frequent malignancy in females, representing 30 percent of all cancers (see Figure 21.1). It is estimated that 180,200 new cases of breast cancer will be diagnosed during 1997 (down from 184,300 new cases in 1996) and that 43,900 women will die from such tumors this year (Ref 119). This is the first time in the 60 years that the American Cancer Society has been keeping national statistics that the number of new cases is expected to decrease, and the second year in a row that the number of deaths from carcinoma of the breast is expected to decrease, a decline from 46,000 deaths in 1995.

The incidence of breast cancer increases throughout a female's life until past age 85; and one out of every eight women living to age 90 will develop carcinoma of the breast.

It is becoming more evident that there is no increased risk of breast cancer in estrogen users.

Research

Studies of both endometrial and breast cancers in estrogen users have indicated a modest association between unopposed estrogen therapy and adenocarcinoma of the endometrium. However, in every instance, the association between estrogen and carcinoma of the breast was considerably less (Ref 51).

The new technique of meta-analysis evaluates multiple studies regarding hormone use and breast cancer. Of the six meta-analyses published, five observed no increased risk of breast cancer from long-term estrogen use, especially when 0.625 mg daily or less of conjugated estrogens were used (Ref 9, 25, 38, 139). One meta-analysis, after rejecting several studies for various reasons (including all follow-up studies), concluded from 16 studies that after 15 years of estrogen use, the relative risk (RR) for breast cancer was 1.3; 95 percent confidence interval (CI), 1.2 to 2.6 (Ref 145). It was stated in the abstract that the increase in risk was largely due to studies that included premenopausal women or women using estradiol. Most of the 16 studies analyzed did not extend 15 years. After eliminating all studies showing a decreased risk, the risk each year was mathematically extrapolated out to 15 years to arrive at the 1.3 RR, an assumption shown not to be true (Ref 24).

At least 55 studies have looked into the relationship
of hormone replacement and breast cancer (Ref 57).
Of the studies observing a significantly increased risk of breast cancer, the increased risk was in different subgroups of estrogen users but not their total patient population (Ref 81, 84, 130).

In the study from Leisure World, the only significantly increased risk of breast cancer (RR=2.5) was in a subgroup of estrogen users with intact ovaries using a total dosage greater than 1,500 mg (Ref 130). In the estrogen users with bilateral oophorectomies, a decreased RR of 0.7 was observed in those using more than 1,500 mg. In the study from England, the significantly increased risk of breast cancer in estrogen users was attributed to the subgroup using high dosages of ethinyl estradiol (Ref 81).

The Nurses' Health Study was the first and only epidemiologic study to observe an overall increased risk of breast cancer in estrogen users (RR=1.32; 95 percent CI, 1.14 to 1.54) (Ref 24). However, there were problems with this study. Detection bias was present in that estrogen users had 14-percent higher screening mammograms than nonusers. They excluded *in situ* carcinoma; but, since 1988, *in situ* cancers have been increasing, while invasive lesions are declining. They also excluded two very important risk factors: alcohol use (RR=2.0) and body mass (RR=1.5). Either one of these risk factors could have accounted for the RR of 1.32.

Additionally, some of the findings in the Nurses' Health Study are not biologically probable. The researchers observed the same increased risk between five and 10 years of estrogen use (RR=1.46; 95 percent CI, 1.22 to 1.75) as was observed with 10 or more years of estrogen use (RR=1.46; 95 percent CI, 1.20 to 1.76). Within two years after discontinuing estrogen replacement, all risks were gone (RR=0.9; 95 percent CI, 0.77 to 1.05). This is just not biologically plausible, since cancers are tumors out of control. Even if the initiating factor was removed (i.e., estrogen), these cancers would keep on growing.

Most studies either failed to find an increased risk of breast cancer, while several observed nonsignificant decreases. A multicenter study did not observe any increased risk of breast cancer in estrogen users, even when taken for many years or the distant past (RR=0.9; 95 percent CI, 0.7 to 1.1) (Ref 89). However, they found significantly decreased risks in three different subgroups of estrogen users, namely, those with:

- Family histories of breast cancer (RR=0.2; 95 percent CI, 0.0 to 0.6)
- First term pregnancies before age 20 (RR=0.1; 95 percent CI, 0.0 to 0.4)
- Parity of one to four (RR=0.6; 95 percent CI, 0.4 to 0.9)

Estrogen-Progestogen Users

The most consistently statistically significant decrease in a subgroup of estrogen users has been observed in those also prescribed a progestogen. Four of the six studies evaluating estrogen-progestogen use found a significant decrease in risk of breast cancer compared to never-users or placebo-treated controls (Ref 53, 91, 108, 144). During the nine years of study and follow-up at Wilford Hall from 1975 to 1983, the lowest incidence of mammary malignancy was significantly decreased in the estrogen-progestogen users to an incidence of 66.8 per 100,000 women (RR=0.3; 95 percent CI, 0.1 to 0.8) (see Table 21.1). There was a nonsignificant decrease in the unopposed estrogen users, with an incidence of 141.0 per 100,000 (RR=0.7; 95 percent CI, 0.5 to 1.1) (see Figure 21.2).

A study from Seattle observed no increased risk of breast cancer with any measure of estrogen use (RR=0.9; 95 percent CI, 0.7 to 1.3) (Ref 144). This was also the first epidemiologic study to confirm the three previous prospective studies that, with more than eight years of estrogen-progestogen use, there was a 60-percent decreased risk of breast cancer (RR=0.4; 95 percent CI, 0.2 to 1.0).

Both the Swedish and Danish studies observed nonsignificantly increased risks of breast cancer in estrogen-progestogen users (RR=4.4; 95 percent CI, 0.9 to 22.4 [Ref 11] and RR=1.36; 95 percent CI, 0.98 to 1.87 [Ref 45]). The Swedish study was based on only 10 patients with six to nine years of estrogen-progestogen use (Ref 11). In fact, in an update of this study by adding four more years of follow-up and six more cases of breast cancer for a total of 16, the RR dropped from 4.4 to 1.3; 95 percent CI, 1.1 to 1.6 (Ref 121). It was not until the ninth and 10th years of ever increasing addition of progestogen to estrogen replacement therapy that a decreased incidence of breast cancer was observed in the Wilford Hall studies (see Figure 21.3).

Improved Prognosis of Breast Cancer in Estrogen Users

In the same month that the Swedish study was published purporting to show an increased risk of breast cancer in hormone users, this same group published another paper utilizing the same database in which it observed a significantly lower mortality rate in breast cancer patients who had received hormone replacement (RR=0.68; 95 percent CI, 0.52 to 0.87) (Ref 10). The report confirmed several other studies, with none to the contrary, indicating an improved prognosis for breast cancer developing in estrogen users (Ref 16, 51, 76, 81, 91, 160).

Burch et al. were the first to observe a 25-percent reduction in mortality from breast cancer when the malignancy developed in estrogen users followed for 15 years (Ref 16). In studies of 256 postmenopausal women with breast cancer, the mortality was 22.2 percent in the 63 hormone users compared to a death rate of 45.5 percent in the 165 nonusers, which was statistically significant with $P \leq 0.005$ (Ref 51).

In a study from England of 4,544 hormone users, the mortality from breast cancer was significantly reduced (RR=0.55; 95 percent CI, 0.28 to 0.96) (Ref 81). With eight to 18 years' follow-up of the 256 patients with breast cancer in the Wilford Hall studies, life table analysis produced median survival times of 84 months for never-users, 80 months for past users, and more than 143 months for current users of estrogen ($P \leq 0.01$) (Ref 147). This study also observed that significantly more of the current estrogen users had positive progesterone receptors (64.7 percent) than nonusers (28 percent) with $P \leq 0.05$.

A large prospective study of 422,373 post-menopausal women by the American Cancer Society showed that ever-use of estrogen replacement therapy was associated with a significantly decreased risk of fatal breast cancer (RR=0.84; 95 percent CI, 0.75 to 0.94) (Ref 160). With six to 10 years of use, the risk was even lower (RR=0.6; 95 percent CI, 0.44 to 0.83).

Recommendations

It is becoming increasingly clear that estrogen therapy does not increase the risk of breast cancer and that the prognosis is improved when carcinoma of the breast develops in hormone users. In addition to a significantly lower incidence of mammary malignancy in estrogen-progestogen users, long-term progesterone deficiency may increase the risk for breast cancer. In a long-term follow-up of a group of infertility patients, those with progesterone deficiency had 5.4 times the risk of premenopausal carcinoma of the breast compared to women in the nonhormone group (Ref 29). The incidence of postmenopausal breast cancer did not differ significantly between the two groups. However, these patients were just reaching menopause. Other studies have observed an increased risk of postmenopausal breast cancer (Ref 28, 102). Chronic anovulation increased the risk of endometrial cancer five-fold, and the risk for breast cancer after the age of 55 was increased to 3.6-fold (Ref 28). Therefore, all postmenopausal women receiving estrogen replacement should also be given progestogens even if they have had hysterectomies.

Our studies have been confirmed by the 22-year study by Nachtigall et al. (Ref 109) in 1992 and the 20-year study by Lauritzen (Ref 90) in 1993. In the longest prospective and follow-up study to date, there were no breast cancers during 22 years in the 116 estrogen-progestogen users while six developed in the 52 never users, which was significant with $P \leq 0.01$ (Ref 109). In the 20-year prospective study from Germany, the incidence of breast cancer in the estrogen-progestogen users was 123.4 per 100,000 compared to 154.6 per 100,000 in the never users, which was significant with $P \leq 0.05$ (Ref 90).

The Seattle study observed that, with more than eight years of estrogen-progestogen use, the risk of carcinoma of the breast was decreased by 60 percent (RR=0.4; 95 percent CI, 0.2 to 1.0) (Ref 144).

Why Progestogens Should Decrease Breast Cancer Risk

Comparative trials between tamoxifen and either medroxyprogesterone acetate or megestrol acetate indicate that progestogens are just as effective in the treatment of metastatic breast cancer (Ref 17). One of the most effective therapies for stage IV metastatic carcinoma of the breast at MD Anderson Cancer Center is a combination of estrogen and progestogen (Ref 80). Seven days of estrogen are given to enhance progesterone receptors in metastatic mammary cancer cells, followed by high-dose medroxyprogesterone acetate for 21 days in repeated cycles. The objective remission response was 56.7 percent for up to six years. Not only do oral contraceptives significantly reduce the risk of benign breast disease but either birth control pills or progestogens reverse both intraductal hyperplasia and atypia of the breast (Ref 157). Performing mastectomy during the luteal phase of the menstrual cycle, when progesterone levels are highest, improves overall survival and recurrence-free interval for breast cancer in premenopausal women (Ref 6, 136, 156).

In a study from France, patients were treated with percutaneous application to the breast for 13 days before surgery with a placebo gel, a gel containing progesterone, or a gel containing estradiol (Ref 20). The mitotic index was significantly lower in the progesterone gel group (0.04) than either the placebo gel group (0.10) or the estradiol gel group (0.20).

In a study of human breast cancer cells in tissue culture, growth fraction was slightly stimulated (13 to 40 percent) with either estradiol or progesterone; however, estradiol plus progesterone significantly reduced growth fraction in 85 percent (Ref 85).

An Australian study of 90 patients with breast cancer treated with continuous combined low-dose estrogen (conjugated estrogens 0.625 mg) and moderate-dose progestogen (medroxyprogesterone acetate 50 mg) observed no deaths in the hormone replacement therapy users, while 9.86 percent of the control group died from breast cancer (Ref 40). A second part of this study, in which 68 subjects were matched with three controls, each in a case control study, confirmed significantly fewer recurrences in the hormone users, seven percent compared to 17 percent of the non-users (RR=0.4; 95 percent CI, 0.17 to 0.93).

Estrogen Use in Breast Cancer Survivors

With the earlier diagnosis and improved prognosis of breast carcinoma, many women are surviving for years after treatment. If estrogens do not increase the risk of mammary malignancy and survival is improved when cancer develops in estrogen users, why not give estrogens to breast cancer survivors? It has always been considered a contraindication, that estrogen therapy would hasten recurrences and increase mortality. There are no data to support this; however, there are also very sparse data to suggest that estrogen therapy is safe.

Several physicians, particularly gynecologic oncologists, have been advocating estrogen replacement therapy in women with previous breast cancer (Ref 35, 146). Now the medical oncologists are joining in this recommendation (Ref 23). While the definitive prospective studies are being done to show that estrogens are safe, which may take 10 to 20 years, there are some preliminary data to suggest its safety. The Australian study observed no deaths and significantly less recurrences in estrogen-progestogen users compared to controls (Ref 40).

Surgeons from southern California reported their experience with 25 women previously treated for breast cancer who subsequently received hormone replacement therapy for 24 to 82 months (Ref 159). There were three recurrences and one death, but the overall survival in this short-term study was 96 percent. In 77 breast cancer survivors given hormone replacement therapy by gynecologic oncologists for up to 15 years (median duration 27 months), there were seven recurrences and three deaths (Ref 35). Therefore, hormone replacement therapy should be discussed with breast cancer survivors since the benefits should outweigh the risks.

TABLE 21.1 – **Incidence of Breast Cancer at Wilford Hall USAF Medical Center: 1975-1983**

THERAPY GROUP	PATIENT-YEARS OF OBSERVATION	PATIENTS WITH CANCER	INCIDENCE (PER 100,000)
Estrogen-Progestogen Users	16,466	11	66.8
Unopposed Estrogen Users	19,676	28	142.3
Estrogen Vaginal Cream Users	4,298	5	116.3
Progestogen Users	1,825	3	164.4
Non-Users	6,404	22	343.5
TOTAL	48,669	69	141.8

FIGURE 21.1—**Incidence of Cancer**

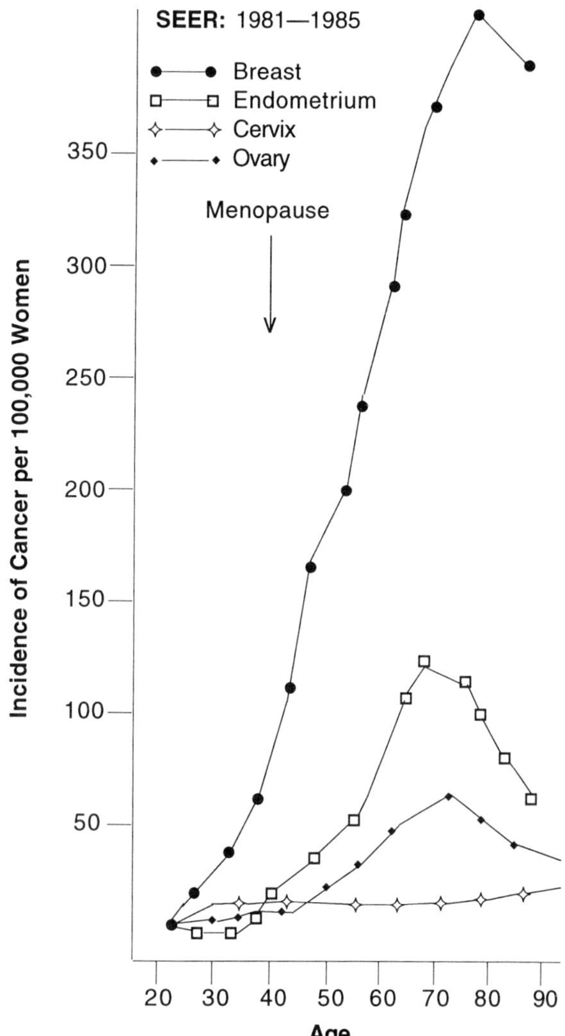

FIGURE 21.1—Incidence of breast, endometrial, cervical, and ovarian cancer in women by age.

FIGURE 21.2—**Incidence of Breast Cancer**

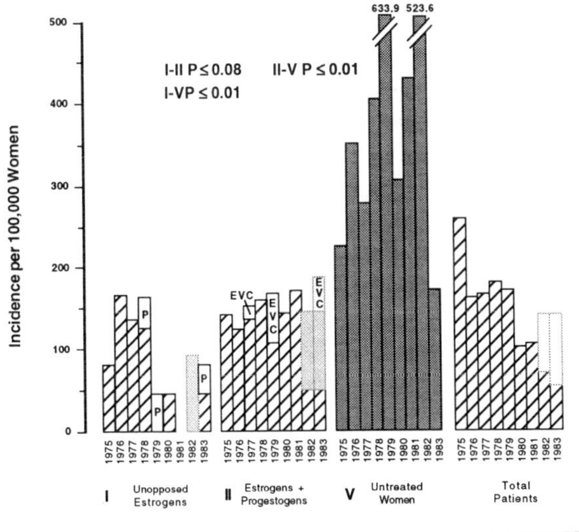

FIGURE 21.2 – Incidence of breast cancer in the various treatment groups compared with untreated from 1975-1983 (Reproduced with permission from Gambrell) (Ref 53).

FIGURE 21.3 – **Incidence of Breast Cancer Compared to Number of Estrogen and Estrogen-Progestogen Treated Women**

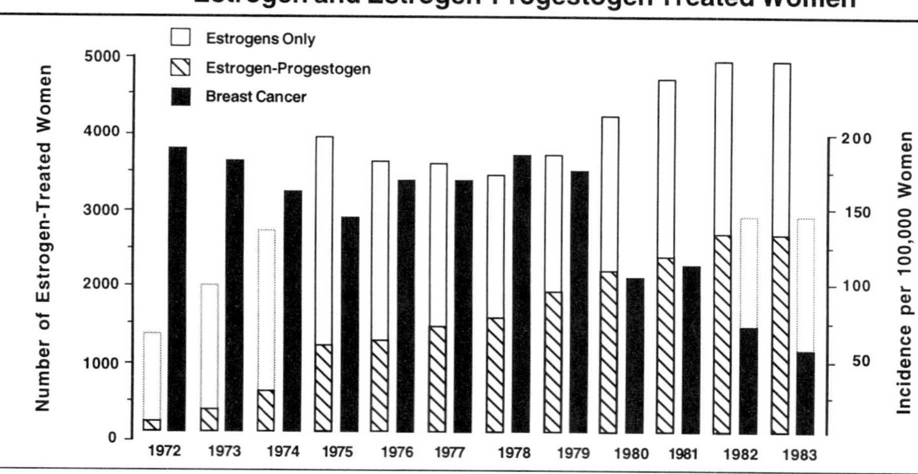

FIGURE 21.3– Comparison of the number of estrogen and estrogen-progestogen users with the incidence of breast cancer by year over the period 1972-1983. Solid lines indicate prospective and follow-up study and broken lines illustrate retrospective data, while semi-broken lines (1982-1983) indicate cancer in past users. (Reproduced with permission from Gambrell) (Ref 53).

NOTES

#22 Thromboembolic Disease

Clinical Information

Estrogen replacement therapy has been thought to increase thromboembolic phenomena, which are listed as contraindications. This concept is largely based on observations suggesting an association between oral contraceptives and vascular thrombosis. Despite a positive association between aging and thromboembolic complications, clinical studies have failed to observe any increased risk of these disorders (Ref 16, 108, 114).

Coagulation changes that occur with aging include:

- Increase in factor V
- Increase in factor VII
- Possible increase in factor VIII
- No change in antithrombin III

Coagulation changes that occur with estrogen replacement include:

- Increase in fibrinogen (still within normal range)
- Slight decrease in antithrombin III (still within normal range)
- Decrease in factor V
- No change in factors VII or X
- No change in prothrombin time or partial thromboplastin time

Research

In one study, deaths from cerebral vascular accidents (CVA) declined from an expected 15 to eight during estrogen therapy over a 15-year period of treatment (Ref 16). It was concluded that estrogens delay aging of the arteries.

In the most recent study, protection from stroke was observed in all age groups except the youngest

(RR=0.53; 95 percent CI, 0.31 to 0.91) (Ref 117). This was unaffected by possible confounding variables such as:

- Smoking
- Alcohol intake
- Body mass
- Exercise

Another study found a significantly lower incidence of stroke syndromes in long-term estrogen users compared with a similar group who had not used estrogens (Ref 72). No significant difference in the incidence of either thrombophlebitis or embolism was observed between estrogen-treated women and patients who had never received estrogens. In a double-blind study, thrombophlebitis occurred in 13 of 84 estrogen-progestogen users and 17 of 84 placebo users (Ref 108). Only one incidence of pulmonary embolism was encountered during the 10 years of this study, and it occurred in a placebo user.

Estrogen labeling has been recently changed so that no longer are all thromboembolic events contraindications. Active thrombophlebitis or thromboembolic disorders remain contraindications as do histories of thrombophlebitis, thrombosis, or thromboembolic disorders associated with previous estrogen use. No longer are postpartum, postoperative, or traumatic blood clots contraindications. However, in patients with any history of thromboembolic disease, it would seem prudent to obtain coagulation studies before therapy and repeat these after three to six months of estrogen use.

#23 Hypertension

Research

Because the original high-dose oral contraceptives caused transient hypertension in some young women, estrogen replacement therapy has been expected to have a similar effect. However, numerous studies have indicated that estrogen therapy has a beneficial effect on hypertension.

Some of these studies and their findings include:

- Duke University - Incidence of new hypertensive cardiovascular disease of 16.3 percent in estrogen-treated women vs 31.7 percent in nonusers ($P \leq 0.001$) (Ref 72)
- Southern California - Study of 1,496 women (after adjusting for effects of obesity) found estrogen-treated women tended to have lower blood pressure and blood glucose than controls (Ref 7)
- Wilford Hall - Estrogen users had lower diastolic blood pressures (BPs) than other groups; nonusers were more obese ($P \leq 0.05$) (Ref 62)
- Australian studies observed lowered systolic BPs with one natural estrogen (Ogen) and lowered diastolic BPs with another (Premarin) (Ref 164)
- An English study observed that both systolic and diastolic BPs are significantly reduced in women on various regimens of hormone replacement (Ref 94)

Hypertension increases in the age group of postmenopausal women. Therefore, cases will be found among these estrogen users (Ref 113, 155). However, these do not establish the role of estrogens in hypertension. Elevations in BPs can coexist with hormone replacement; therefore, blood pressure should be routinely monitored.

Other studies have reported on the effect of estrogen use on the renin-aldosterone system. One study showed no activation of the renin-aldosterone system in patients using estradiol valerate therapy (Ref 126). Another study reported an increased plasma renin activity in users of conjugated estrogens but no effect on the renin concentration itself (Ref 118). Neither study observed any adverse effect of estrogens on blood pressures when hormone users were matched to controls and corrected for age and weight.

Recommendations for Treatment

If hypertension does occur in estrogen users, estrogen replacement does not have to stop (Ref 126). Instead, as a step, salt intake should be restricted to 3,000 mg daily. If salt restriction alone does not control the hypertension, a mild antihypertensive, such as hydrochlorothiazide at 25 to 50 mg daily, can be added. Only if these two measures fail to improve blood pressure levels should there be consideration of ending estrogen replacement. Most hypertensive patients require less medication after hormone replacement.

#24 Gallbladder Disease

Research

Some studies have indicated that estrogen replacement therapy increases the risk of gallbladder disease, especially cholelithiasis. The liver responds to oral estrogens by an increase in sex hormone binding globulin (SHBG). It has been suggested that oral estrogens may affect the liver's excretory functions and increase the incidence of gallstones.

Gallstones seem to occur more frequently in the silent form. In one study, oral cholecystography showed that 5.1 percent of those tested had gallstones present (Ref 131). Silent cases occurred twice as often, and the diet was not significantly different in those with or without gallstones.

One evaluative study reported that the risk of surgically confirmed gallbladder disease increased 2.5 times with estrogen therapy (Ref 13). In another study, the risk of cholesterol cholelithiasis was increased by both estrogens and obesity (Ref 79). Both factors operated independently, with estrogen increasing the risk of gallstones at all weight levels. However, in the Duke University study, new occurrence of gallbladder disease was significantly lower ($P \leq 0.05$) in the estrogen users compared with controls (Ref 72). At the end of a 10-year New York study, the estrogen-progestogen group had a higher, although statistically insignificant, incidence of cholelithiasis (Ref 108).

The most recent study found no increased risk for gallstones among estrogen users (RR=1.18; 95 percent CI, 0.65 to 2.13) (Ref 86). Among estrogen users, the duration of use was similar in cases and controls.

Recommendations for Treatment

Since it is not feasible to screen all postmenopausal women for occult gallbladder disease prior to estrogen therapy, it has been suggested that patients should be instructed regarding the early signs of cholelithiasis (Ref 79), including:

- Right upper quadrant pain
- Indigestion
- Eructation
- Nausea

24.

#25 Nutrition and Diet

A healthy lifestyle is very important for postmenopausal women. Remaining active, not smoking, choosing the right foods, and not gaining weight help prevent cardiovascular diseases and decrease other problems of aging. Estrogen replacement therapy, as important as it is, should not be a substitute for a healthy lifestyle.

Body Weight

It is commonly thought that menopause, estrogen therapy, and even hysterectomy cause women to gain weight. This is just not true. What happens to cause some women to gain weight is that, at menopause, metabolism decreases. Some cannot continue to eat the same this year as last year because of decreased metabolism.

In the recently published, three-year PEPI trial (Ref 165), in 875 healthy postmenopausal women, all patients gained weight. The greatest weight gain was in the placebo group, which had an average weight gain of 4.6 pounds, compared to the estrogen user group, which had an average weight gain of 1.5 pounds.

A healthy lifestyle becomes even more important after menopause. Smoking decreases the good HDL cholesterol, which aids in removal of cholesterol from the blood. Increased activity, such as long, brisk walks, increases HDL cholesterol. Strategies for keeping cholesterol low and remaining healthy are to:

- Reduce the amount of total and saturated fat and cholesterol in the diet
- Use monounsaturated oils instead of saturated fats
- Eat foods high in soluble fiber, e.g., oat bran

- Eat foods high in beta carotene and other antioxidants
- Drink coffee in moderation
- Limit the amount of salt in the diet
- Eat calcium-rich foods (see Section #18)

Fat Grams

Counting calories from fat is not only most important for losing and maintaining weight but also is the best diet method for lowering cholesterol and triglyceride levels. This recent advance has been a major breakthrough in weight reduction. Calories from fat grams are far more important than total calories in the diet. For women, restricting the diet to no more than 20 to 25 fat grams per day can result in a one- to three-pound weight loss each week. The T-Factor Diet (Ref 88) is an excellent source for determining fat grams in foods and recipes and general instructions on how to lose and maintain weight.

#26 Lipid Metabolism

Changes in Blood Lipid Profile

Both surgical and natural menopause appear to be related to adverse changes in blood lipid profile. These changes include:

- Development of atherosclerosis at an earlier age
- Increased hypertension
- Increased incidence of coronary artery disease

Natural Estrogens

Low dosages of natural estrogens increase HDL cholesterol with corresponding decreases in both LDL and very low density lipoproteins (VLDL), an antiatherogenic pattern.

Transdermal estradiol and subcutaneous estradiol pellets also increase HDL cholesterol, but seem to take longer than oral estrogens because they avoid the first liver-pass. In a comparative study between estradiol pellets and transdermal estradiol, there was a significant increase in HDL cholesterol with the pellets after 12 weeks; it took 24 weeks for the patch to increase HDL significantly (Ref 143). The total cholesterol-to-HDL ratio was also significantly decreased at 12 weeks with pellets but took 24 weeks with the patch.

In the Coronary Drug Project, high dosages of conjugated estrogens (5 to 15 mg) had the opposite effect of lower dosages, resulting in an atherogenic pattern of decreased HDL with corresponding increases of both LDL and VLDL (Ref 27).

FIGURE 26.1 — Changes in Lipoproteins

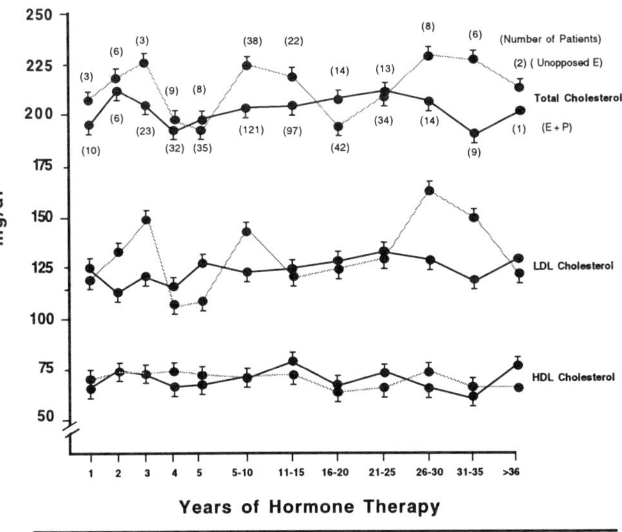

Mean values of total cholesterol, LDL cholesterol, and HDL cholesterol compared in the unopposed estrogen users (unopposed E) to the estrogen-progestogen users (E + P) from one to 44 years of hormone replacement therapy. (Reproduced from Gambrell and Teran with permission of the publisher) (Ref 64).

Birth Control Pills

Moderate-to-high dosage oral contraceptives, e.g., 50 mg of ethinyl estradiol, increase both HDL and VLDL. However, when the 19-nor-testosterone progestogens are added, the atherogenic pattern develops with a decrease in HDL, while LDL and VLDL both increase. HDL is further decreased by smoking and results in a relative risk of 2.5 for heart disease mortality (Ref 101). The newer low-dosage oral contraceptives do not have an adverse effect on lipid metabolism.

Added Progestogens

Although natural estrogens increase HDL cholesterol, concern has been expressed that added progestogens may negate this beneficial effect. Most of this concern is based on short-term studies of estrogen-progestogen use that have not been confirmed in studies of more than 12 months' duration (Ref 8, 83).

In one such study (Ref 8):

- HDL was significantly increased and LDL significantly decreased in both unopposed estrogen users and estrogen-progestogen users
- Triglycerides were significantly increased in unopposed estrogen users but not different from controls in estrogen-progestogen users

This shows that added progestogens may actually benefit the lipid pattern by minimizing the increase in triglycerides usually seen with estrogen therapy. This was confirmed in a large study of 4,958 postmenopausal women where it was also observed that estrogen users had higher levels of apolipoprotein A-1 than nonusers (Ref 106).

Another study evaluated different dosages of Estrace using a standard dosage of progestogen, 1 mg of norethindrone acetate for 11 days (Ref 83). The study found:

- A dose-related increase in HDL
- 4 mg ↑ HDL <2 mg <1 mg Estrace
- Significant decrease in LDL with all three dosages
- Norethindrone acetate did not negate the increase in HDL or decrease in LDL

The three-year PEPI trail (Ref 165) concluded that estrogen alone or in combination with the progestogen improves lipoprotein levels and lowers fibrinogen levels without detectable effects on postchallenge insulin or blood pressure. Unopposed estrogen produced the greatest increase in HDL cholesterol, but there was a high incidence of endometrial hyperplasia. Conjugated estrogens with cyclic medroxyprogesterone acetate had the most favorable effect on HDL cholesterol without any risk of endometrial hyperplasia.

Over the long-term there are no adverse effects on lipids of added progestogens to estrogen replacement. In a long-term study, the only significant changes were related to obesity (↑ triglycerides) and smoking (↓ HDL) (Ref 64). In this cross-sectional study at the Medical College of Georgia:

- 556 were postmenopausal women
- 132 were using unopposed estrogen
- 424 were using estrogen and progestogen
- The age range was 44 to 85 years, with a mean age of 57.14 ± 10.56 years
- Duration of therapy was from one to 44 years, with a mean duration of 11.97 ± 8.11 years

Figure 26.1 shows the mean values from one to more than 36 years of hormone replacement. Total cholesterol hovered around 200 to 210 mg/dL in both unopposed estrogen users and estrogen-progestogen users. LDL ranged from 110 to 130 mg/dL in both groups (normal range 86 to 138). There were no differences in mean HDL, ranging from 60 to 70 mg/dL (average risk 54 to 59; low risk 59 to 74). There were no significant differences in mean HDL among unopposed estrogen users (67.0 ± 3.94), estrogen plus C-21 progestogen users (64.5 ± 4.16), and estrogen plus C-19 progestogen users (61.9 ± 3.84).

Even androgens do not adversely affect lipids when adequate dosages of estrogen are given, since 84.2 percent of these patients also received androgens, usually in the form of testosterone pellets.

The tremendous benefit of preventing cardiovascular disease with hormone replacement therapy cannot be fully explained by the changes in lipid patterns (Ref 132). Other factors have roles such as direct effects of estrogens on arterial walls, since estrogen receptors have been identified in coronary vessels.

Estrogens may:

- Improve vascular blood flow, even dilatation of coronary arteries
- Decrease platelet adhesiveness
- Increase endothelial-derived relaxing factor (EDRF)
- Be mediated through prostacyclin and thromboxane metabolism
- Increase cardiac output
- Reduce vascular resistance
- Increase velocity of blood flow
- Inhibit atherosclerosis progression
- Inhibit coronary thrombosis

NOTES

#27 Management of Side Effects

Resumption of Menses

In postmenopausal women treated with combination estrogen-progestogen therapy, withdrawal bleeding occurs in as many as 97 percent until age 60, decreasing to 60 percent after age 65.

Generally, patient acceptance of resumption of menses has been good if the relative benefits and risks are carefully explained. These include:

- The reduced incidence of endometrial cancer (see Section #20)
- No increased risk of breast cancer; in some women, added progestogen reduces its incidence (see Section #21)
- Promotion of new bone formation, helping restore bone that has been lost to osteoporosis (see Section #5)

In addition, the menses often change for the better. Frequently, the menses:

- Are lighter
- Are less painful
- Have less abnormal bleeding

Patients most reluctant to resume menses are those who experienced adverse menstrual effects. After menopause, withdrawal menses from hormone therapy are usually:

- Only three to four days in duration
- Free of dysmenorrhea
- Without premenstrual syndrome (PMS) symptoms

In one study (Ref 60), abnormal bleeding requiring curettage occurred in:

- 23.3 percent of nonusers of hormones
- 14 percent of unopposed estrogen users
- Only 3.9 percent of estrogen-progestogen users

In addition, the estrogen-progestogen users need not have the annual endometrial biopsies that are recommended for all unopposed estrogen users with intact uteri (see Section #10).

For those patients who cannot tolerate resumption of menses, cyclic combined estrogen-progestogen therapy is an alternative that will produce amenorrhea in 75 percent of patients after four to six months (see Section #16).

Side Effects of Estrogens

Side effects of estrogens may include:

- Breast tenderness
- Edema or bloating
- PMS-like symptoms
- Nausea
- Headaches

Most patients have few, if any, side effects from estrogen replacement. If side effects occur, they are minimal and transient (Ref 56).

Breast tenderness and sometimes slight breast enlargement may occur during the first two to three months after initiation of therapy. Mastodynia usually abates with time, and reassurance is often all that patients need.

If breast tenderness persists, the estrogen dosage can be reduced if more than 0.625 mg conjugated estrogens were prescribed. However, this should be the lowest dosage in order to prevent osteoporosis (see Section #5).

Adding a progestogen to estrogen therapy reduces breast tenderness in time, although it may initially aggravate breast tenderness. Reassurance to patients is often all that is needed. Adding androgens to estrogen therapy or to estrogen-progestogen therapy may also ameliorate breast tenderness.

A mild diuretic, such as hydrochlorothiazide or spironolactone (25 to 50 mg), will relieve symptoms caused by estrogen-related fluid retention, such as:

- Edema
- Bloating
- Abdominal pressure
- Breast tenderness
- PMS-like symptoms (headache, irritability)

The diuretic is usually given seven to 10 days before menses during the days of added progestogen. A change to a different estrogen is sometimes necessary (see Table 13.1) or a change in the route of administration, e.g., the transdermal estrogen, may help.

Nausea is rare in the low dosages of estrogen usually required for estrogen replacement. If nausea persists after two months of therapy, a change of estrogens or the route of administration may help.

Headaches are generally relieved by estrogen replacement. Most headaches are transient and respond to analgesics. Others may occur only with cyclic therapy on the days at the end of the month when estrogens are not taken. Estrogens can be taken continuously as long as they are opposed with progestogens for 13 days each month. Usually, migraine headaches diminish at menopause and sometimes recur with estrogen replacement. Sometimes headaches respond to a mild diuretic, but it may be necessary to add an androgen to the estrogen therapy. The best response is offered by combination products such as:

- Estratest (orally)
- Depo-Testadiol (by injection)
- Estradiol-testosterone pellets

Side Effects of Progestogens

Side effects of progestogens include:

- PMS-like symptoms
- Lethargy
- Depression and irritability
- Abdominal bloating
- Breast tenderness

Mild PMS-like symptoms usually respond to a diuretic such as hydrochlorothiazide or spironolactone at 25 to 50 mg for seven to 10 days before menses. If this is ineffective, a change should be made to another oral progestogen.

Breast tenderness may be initiated, aggravated, or relieved when progestogens are added to estrogen replacement. Symptoms usually abate after three to six months. If mastodynia persists, a change should be made to another progestogen (see Table 16.1).For some women, C-21 progestogens such as medroxyprogesterone acetate are better than 19-nor-testosterone progestogens such as norethindrone acetate. For others, the reverse is true.

In a rare case, a woman may experience side effects with all oral progestogens. Progesterone vaginal suppositories (25 to 50 mg) or oral micronized progesterone (100 to 300 mg) often eliminate these reactions.

#28 Contraindications

Contraindications for Estrogens

The following contraindications are listed in the product literature for most estrogens:

- Known or suspected cancer of the breast
- Known or suspected estrogen-dependent neoplasia
- Known or suspected pregnancy
- Undiagnosed abnormal genital bleeding
- Active thrombophlebitis or thromboembolic disorders

Women on estrogen replacement therapy have not been reported to have an increased risk of thrombophlebitis and/or thromboembolic disease. However, there is insufficient information regarding women who have had previous thromboembolic disease.

There is no evidence that estrogen replacement increases the risk for breast cancer. However, estrogen is the growth hormone of mammary tissue, and contraindications should be observed for medical and/ or legal reasons until further data are accumulated (see Section #21).

Four prominent gynecologic oncologists now recommend that patients with successfully treated breast cancer be allowed to use hormone replacement, since there are no data indicating it worsens prognosis (Ref 35, 40, 146). Theoretically, estrogen receptors in carcinoma of the breast would allow selection of some patients for estrogen replacement, yet only 50 percent of estrogen receptor positive tumors will respond either to endocrine ablative surgery or antiestrogen therapy. When progesterone receptors in mammary cancer are also positive, this predictive response increases to 70 percent.

Endometrial cancer may not have to remain a strict contraindication. Gynecologic oncologists at Wilford Hall USAF Medical Center provided estrogen replacement in women with Stage I well differentiated adenocarcinoma of the endometrium, since there was little likelihood of metastases. The five-year survival rate was in excess of 96.7 percent. A study from Duke University indicated that prognosis was actually improved in endometrial cancer patients treated with estrogens (Ref 31).

Any abnormal postmenopausal bleeding should be thoroughly evaluated (see Section #10). Once malignancy is excluded and endometrial hyperplasia has been adequately treated with progestogens (see Section #19), estrogen-progestogen therapy can be safely administered.

Although there is no evidence that low dosages of natural estrogens have any adverse effects on coagulation factors or thromboembolic disease (see Section #22), estrogen replacement should be given cautiously to women who had blood clots previously while using estrogens. Thromboembolic events not related to a history of hormone use no longer are contraindications for replacement therapy.

Contraindications for Progestogens

The following contraindications are listed in the product literature for most progestogens:

- A past or present history of:
  - Thrombophlebitis
  - Thromboembolic disorders
  - Cerebral apoplexy 28.
- Liver dysfunction or disease
- Known or suspected carcinoma of the breast
- Undiagnosed vaginal bleeding
- Missed abortion
- As a diagnostic test for pregnancy

Almost identical contraindications are listed for progestogens as for estrogens, even though there is no evidence that progestogens have any adverse effect on coagulation factors or thromboembolic disorders. However, this labeling should not preclude physicians from using their best judgments in the interest of their patients.

If liver function studies are normal, patients with histories of liver dysfunction or disease can safely be given progestogens. However, liver function studies should be repeated after three to six months of progestogen therapy.

There is no evidence that progestogens increase the risk for breast cancer. There is, in fact, increasing evidence that adding progestogens to estrogen replacement may decrease the risk for carcinoma of the breast in some women (see Section #21) and that long-term progesterone deficiency can increase the risk for breast cancer (Ref 28, 29). For medical and/or legal reasons, prescribing progestogens for therapies other than for treatment of metastatic carcinoma of the breast (Megace) is hazardous in the U.S.

In addition to Megace, Provera is also used to treat metastatic breast carcinoma in Canada and Europe and is just beginning to be used in the U.S. (Ref 17, 80). Comparative trials between tamoxifen and Provera indicate that progestogens are just as effective in the treatment of metastatic breast cancer as the weak estrogen tamoxifen (Ref 17).

One of the most effective therapies for Stage IV metastatic carcinoma of the breast at the MD Anderson Cancer Center was a combination of estrogen and progestogen (Ref 80). Seven days of estrogen were given to enhance progesterone receptors in mammary cancer cells, followed by 21 days of high-dose Provera for 21 days in repeated cycles. The objective remission response was 56.7 percent for up to six years, with a mean duration of 22 months. Yet it is ironic that this progestogen, as well as all other progestogens except Megace, remain listed as contraindicated for women with breast cancer in the U.S.

Undiagnosed genital bleeding becomes apparent in the course of proper evaluation of postmenopausal women (see Section #10). Endometrial hyperplasia should be treated with progestogens to prevent adenocarcinoma of the endometrium.

#29 Alternative Therapy

Clinical Information

Estrogens and progestogens are always the preferred hormone replacement treatment since they:

- Relieve menopausal symptoms
- Prevent the metabolic consequences (osteoporosis and atherosclerosis) of long-term estrogen deficiency

If estrogens are contraindicated, progestogens cannot be used since the contraindications are identical (see Section #28). Alternative therapies are available to treat menopausal symptoms, including:

- Vasomotor symptoms
- Urogenital atrophy
- Psychogenic manifestations
- Osteoporosis

Vasomotor Symptoms

Androgens are effective in relieving such symptoms as:

- Hot flushes (or flashes)
- Night sweats
- Psychogenic manifestations

Any of the oral androgens such as methyltestosterone 5 mg (see Table 15.1) or injectables such as Depo-Testosterone (50 mg every four weeks) can be used. However, androgens do not prevent atrophic vaginitis or coronary artery disease, and they are probably ineffective in preventing osteoporosis in the dosages that can be given to postmenopausal women.

Bellergal-S (by Sandoz) is a tablet combining phenobarbital, ergotamine, and belladonna alkaloids given in a dosage of one tablet twice daily. It is effective for:

- Reducing hot flushes
- Reducing night sweats
- Helping to calm restlessness
- Relieving insomnia

Clonidine HCl is an antihypertensive agent effective for hot flushes. The dosage is 0.1 mg three times daily.

Urogenital Atrophy

No good alternative to estrogen is available for treatment of atrophic vaginitis. If oral estrogens are contraindicated, so are estrogen vaginal creams, which are well absorbed through the vaginal mucosa. Local antibiotics will treat infections, and one- to two-percent testosterone cream is effective for kraurosis vulvae.

Surgical lubricants can be prescribed for dyspareunia. Replens Vaginal Moisturizer (Columbia Laboratories) is a new product specifically designed to treat postmenopausal vaginal dryness.

Psychogenic Manifestations

Alternative therapies available for treatment of psychogenic manifestations include:

- Tranquilizers
- Androgens
- Calcium channel blockers

Tranquilizers can be used to treat depression and restlessness, but they are not good substitutes for estrogen replacement since they do not prevent effects of menopausal estrogen deprivation.

Androgens are most effective when they can be prescribed along with estrogens. Used alone, androgens still offer:

- Treatment of disturbances of the libido
- Promotion of a sense of well-being
- Partial relief of depression

A calcium channel blocker (Calan by Searle) can be fairly effective in relieving headaches. It works best when combined with estrogen replacement but can be effective used alone. The dosage is titrated, starting with 80 mg daily and increasing every week to a maximum of four times daily until headaches are blocked.

Osteoporosis and Atherosclerosis

When estrogens are contraindicated, calcium supplementation should be increased to 1,500 to 2,000 mg daily (see Section #18). There is some evidence that calcium alone will help prevent osteoporosis and reduce fracture rate (Ref 44, 127), although this has recently been questioned. It is best to provide estrogen replacement whenever possible.

In addition to these higher doses of calcium, calcitonin is probably the best preventive for osteoporosis when estrogens are contraindicated. However, calcitonin is:

- Expensive
- In short supply, until recently
- Given by injection at least three times weekly

Nasal calcitonin has recently been approved for treatment of osteoporosis (Miacalcin by Sandoz). It may not prevent bone loss in the immediate postmenopausal period, but a reduction in bone loss and fracture rate has been shown in older women (Ref 66, 124). Nasal calcitonin 200 IU used cyclicly (one month on and one month off over two years) increased both spine bone mineral density and stiffness in the oscalcis by two percent (Ref 124).

Bisphosphonates, such as etidronate, seem to be effective in reducing vertebral fractures. However, the long-term effects are unknown, as are its effects on the cortical bone in the hip (see Section #5).

Fosamax (alendronate) is a newly released bisphosphonate that shows more promise. The dosage is 10 mg daily, which must be taken before the first food of the day with a glass of water (Ref 36, 42). It may increase trabecular bone in the spine by five to 10 percent over the first two years and also is effective in reducing hip and wrist fractures. The FDA has just approved Fosamax 5 mg to prevent osteoporosis (see Section #5).

There is really no alternative to estrogen replacement for prevention of atherosclerosis. Good nutrition is advisable to reduce dietary intake of cholesterol (see Section #25). Other measures include increases in physical activities, e.g., jogging or taking brisk walks.

#30 References

1. Adams MR, Washburn SA, Wagner JD, et al: Arterial changes: Estrogen deficiency and effects of hormone replacement. In: Treatment of the Postmenopausal Woman: Basic and Clinical Aspects, RA Lobo (ed). New York, Raven Press, 1994, pp 243-250.

2. American-Canadian Cooperative Study Group: Persantine aspirin trial in cerebral ischemia-Part III: Risk factor for stroke. Stroke 1986;17:12.

3. Anderson E, Hamburger S, Lin JH, et al: Characteristics of menopausal women seeking assistance. Am J Obstet Gynecol 1987;156:428.

4. Annual Cancer Statistics Review. NIH Publication No. 88-2789. Bethesda, National Institutes of Health, 1987, p III. 36.

5. Armstrong BK: Oestrogen therapy after the menopause: Boon or bane? Med J Austral 1988;148:213.

6. Badwe RA, Gregory WN, Chaudry MN, et al: Timing of surgery during menstrual cycle and survival of premenopausal women with operable breast cancer. Lancet 1991;337:1261.

7. Barrett-Conner E, Brown V, Turner J, et al: Heart disease risk factors and hormone use in postmenopausal women. JAMA 1978;241:2167.

8. Barrett-Conner E, Wingard DL, Criqui MH: Postmenopausal estrogen use and heart disease risk factors in the 1980s. JAMA 1989;261:2095.

9. Bates SK: Postmenopausal estrogen replacement therapy and breast cancer. J Soc Obstet Gynaecol Can 1990;12:9.

10. Bergkvist L, Adami H-O, Persson I, et al: Prognosis after breast cancer diagnosis in women exposed to estrogen and estrogen-progestogen replacement therapy. Am J Epidemiol 1989;130:221.

11. Bergkvist L, Adami H-O, Persson I, et al: The risk of breast cancer after estrogen and estrogen-progestin replacement. N Engl J Med 1989;321:293.

12. Birge SJ: The role of estrogen deficiency in the aging central nervous system. In: Treatment of the Postmenopausal Woman: Basic and Clinical Aspects, RA Lobo, (ed). New York, Raven Press, 1994, pp 153-157.

13. Boston Collaborative Drug Surveillance Program: Surgically confirmed gallbladder disease, venous thromboembolism, and breast tumors in relation to postmenopausal estrogen therapy. N Engl J Med 1974;290:15.

14. Brenner DE, Kukull WA, Stergachis A, et al: Postmenopausal estrogen replacement therapy and the risk of Alzheimer's disease: A population-based case-control study. Am J Epidemiol 1994;140:262.

15. Brown KH, Hammond CB: Urogenital atrophy. Obstet Gynecol Clin N Am 1987;15:13.

16. Burch JC, Byrd BF, Vaughn WK: Results of estrogen treatment in one thousand hysterectomized women for 14,318 years. In: Consensus on Menopausal Research. Van Keep PA, Greenblatt RB, Albeaux-Fernet M (eds.) Lancaster, England: MTP Press Ltd., 1976;164.

17. Buzdar AU: Progestins in cancer treatment. In: Endocrine Management of Cancer. Stoll, BA (ed.) Basel, Switzerland: Karger, 1988;1.

18. Campbell S, Whitehead M: Oestrogen therapy and the menopausal syndrome. In: Clinics in Obstetrics and Gynaecology. Greenblatt RB, Studd JWW (eds.) London, England: WB Saunders Co., Ltd., 1977:31.

19. Cedars MI, Judd HL: Non-oral routes of estrogen administration. Obstet Gynecol Clin N Am 1987;14:269.

20. Chang K-J, Lee TTY, Linaras-Cruz et al: Influences of percutaneous administration of estradiol and progesterone on human breast epithelial cells *in vivo*. Fertil Steril 1995;63:785.

21. Chetkowski RJ, Meldrum DR, Steingold KA, et al: Biologic effects of transdermal estradiol. N Engl J Med 1986;314:1615.

22. Christiansen C, Christensen MS, Transbol I: Bone mass in postmenopausal women after withdrawal of oestrogen/progestogen replacement therapy. Lancet 1981;1:459.

23. Cobleigh MA, Berris RF, Bush T, et al: Estrogen replacement therapy in breast cancer survivors: A time for change. JAMA 1994;272:540.

24. Colditz GA, Hankinson SE, Hunter DJ et al: The use of estrogens and progestins and the risk of breast cancer in postmenopausal women. N Engl J Med 1995;332:1589.

25. Colditz GA, Egan KM, Stampfer MJ: Hormone replacement therapy and risk of breast cancer: Results from epidemiologic studies. Am J Obstet Gynecol 1993;168:1473.

26. Comerci JT Jr, Fields AL, Runowitz LD, Goldberg GL: Continuous low-dose combined hormonal replacement therapy and the risk of endometrial cancer. Gynecol Oncol 1997; 64:425.

27. The Coronary Drug Project Research Group: The coronary drug project: Initial findings leading to modifications of its research protocol. JAMA 1970;214:1303.

28. Coulam CB, Annegers JF: Chronic anovulation may increase postmenopausal breast cancer risk. JAMA 1983;249:445.

29. Cowan LD, Gordis L, Tonascia JA, et al: Breast cancer incidence in women with a history of progesterone deficiency. Am J Epidemiol 1981;114:209.

30. Creasman WT: Estrogen replacement therapy: Is previously treated cancer a contraindication? Obstet Gynecol 1991;77:308.

31. Creasman WT, Henderson D, Hindshaw W, et al: Estrogen replacement therapy in the patient treated for endometrial cancer. Obstet Gynecol 1986;67:326.

32. Crilley RG, Marshall DH, Nordin BEC: The effect of oestradiol valerate and cyclic oestradiol valerate/dl-norgestrel on calcium metabolism. Postgrad Med J 1978;54:47.

33. Darj E, Nilsson S, Axelsson O, et al: Clinical and endometrial effects of estradiol and progesterone in postmenopausal women. Maturitas 1991;13:109.

34. Dennerstein L, Laby B, Burrows GD, et al: Headache and sex hormone therapy. Headache 1978;18:146.

35. DeSaia PJ, Creasman WT, Odicino F, et al: Hormone replacement therapy in breast cancer. Lancet 1993;324:1232.

36. Devogelaer JP, Broll H, Correa-Rotter R, et al: Oral alendronate induces progressive increases in bone mass of the spine, hip, and total body over three years in postmenopausal women with osteoporosis. Bone 1996;18:141.

37. Doren M, Schneider HPG: Long-term compliance of continuous combined estrogen and progestogen replacement in postmenopausal women. Maturitas 1996;25:99.

38. Dupont WD, Page DL: Menopausal estrogen replacement therapy and breast cancer. Arch Intern Med 1991;151:67.

39. Ebeling PR, Altey LM, Guthrie JR et al: Bone turnover markers and bone density across the menopausal transition. J Clin Endocr Metab 1996;81:3366.

40. Eden JA, Bush T, Nard S, et al: A case-controlled study of combined continuous estrogen-progestin replacement therapy among women with a personal history of breast cancer: Menopause. J N Am Menopause Soc 1995;2:67.

41. El-Maraghy MA, El-Badawy N, Wafa GA, et al: Progesterone challenge test in postmenopausal women at high risk. Maturitas 1994;19:53.

42. Ensrud K, Black D, Barrett-Conner E et al: Alendronate prevents fractures in women at very high risk: Results from the fracture intervention trial. J Bone Miner Res 1996;11(Suppl 1):s133.

43. Ettinger B, Genant HK, Cann CE: Long-term replacement therapy prevents bone loss and fractures. Ann Intern Med 1985;102:319.

44. Ettinger B, Genant HK, Steiger P, et al: Low-dosage micronized 17á-estradiol prevents bone loss in postmenopausal women. Am J Obstet Gynecol 1992;166:479.

45. Ewertz M: Influence of noncontraceptive exogenous and endogenous sex hormones in breast cancer risks in Denmark. Int J Cancer 1988;42:832.

46. Gallagher JC, Kable WT, Goldgar D: Effect of progestin therapy on cortical and trabecular bone: Comparison with estrogen. Am J Med 1991;90:171.

47. Gallagher JC, Riggs RL, Deluca HF: Effect of estrogen on calcium absorption and serum vitamin D metabolites in postmenopausal osteoporosis. J Clin Metab Endocrinol 1980;51:1359.

48. Gambrell RD Jr: Breast disease in the postmenopausal years. Seminar Reprod Endocrinol 1983;1:27.

49. Gambrell RD Jr: Hormone replacement therapy and breast cancer. Maturitas 1987;9:123.

50. Gambrell RD Jr: Prevention of endometrial cancer with progestogens. Maturitas 1986;8:159.

51. Gambrell RD Jr: Proposal to decrease the risk and improve the prognosis of breast cancer. Am J Obstet Gynecol 1984;150:119.

52. Gambrell RD Jr: Sex steroids and cancer. Obstet Gynecol Clin N Am 1987;14:91.

53. Gambrell RD Jr: Studies of endometrial and breast disease with hormone replacement therapy. In: The Menopause. Studd JWW, Whitehead MI (eds.) Oxford, England: Blackwell Scientific Publication, Ltd., 1988;247-261.

54. Gambrell RD Jr: The menopause: Benefits and risks of estrogen-progestogen replacement therapy. Fertil Steril 1982;37:457.

55. Gambrell RD Jr: Use of progestogen therapy. Am J Obstet Gynecol 1987;156:1304.

56. Gambrell RD Jr: Management of hormone replacement side effects: Menopause. J N Am Menopause Soc 1994;1:67.

57. Gambrell RD Jr: Hormone replacement therapy and breast cancer risk. Arch Fam Med 1996;5:341.

58. Gambrell RD Jr: Strategies to reduce the incidence of endometrial cancer in postmenopausal women. Am J Obstet Gynecol 1997 (in press).

59. Gambrell RD Jr, Cherry JK, Davis DL, et al: (Letter) Mammography screening. JAMA 1994;271:1827.

60. Gambrell RD Jr, Castaneda TA, Ricci CA: Management of postmenopausal bleeding to prevent endometrial cancer. Maturitas 1978;1:99.

61. Gambrell RD Jr, Massey FM, Castaneda TA, et al: Use of the progestogen challenge test to reduce the risk of endometrial cancer. Obstet Gynecol 1980;55:732.

62. Gambrell RD Jr, Maier RC, Sanders BI: Decreased incidence of breast cancer in postmenopausal estrogen-progestogen users. Obstet Gynecol 1983;62:435.

63. Gambrell RD Jr, McDonough PG: The "red queen" and endometrial hyperplasia. Fertil Steril 1994;61:401.

64. Gambrell RD Jr, Teran AZ: Changes in lipids and lipoproteins with long term estrogen deficiency and hormone replacement therapy. Am J Obstet Gynecol 1991; 165:307.

65. Gibbons WE, Moyer DL, Lobo RA, et al: Biochemical and histologic effects of sequential estrogen/progestin therapy on the endometrium of postmenopausal women. Am J Obstet Gynecol 1986;154;456.

66. Gonnelli S, Cepollaro C, Pondrelli C et al: Ultrasound parameters in osteoporotic patients treated with salmon calcitonin: A longitudinal study. Osteoporosis Int 1996;6:303.

67. Goodman L, Awwad J, Marc K, et al: Continuous combined hormonal replacement therapy and the risk of endometrial cancer: Menopause. J N Am Menopause Soc 1994;1:57.

68. Gordon GS: Drug treatment of the osteoporoses. Ann Rev Pharmacol Toxicol 1978;18:253.

69. Greenblatt RB: The use of androgens in the menopause and other gynecic disorders. Obstet Gynecol Clin N Am 1987;14:251.

70. Gruchow HW, Anderson AJ, Barborink JJ, et al: Postmenopausal use of estrogen and occlusion of coronary arteries. Am Heart J 1988;115:954.

71. Gusberg SB: The individual at high risk for endometrial carcinoma. Am J Obstet Gynecol 1976;126:535.

72. Hammond CB, Jelovsek FR, Lee KL, et al: Effects of long-term estrogen replacement therapy: I-Metabolic. Am J Obstet Gynecol 1979;133:525.

73. Hammond CB, Jelovsek FR, Lee KL, et al: Effects of long-term estrogen replacement therapy: II-Neoplasia. Am J Obstet Gynecol 1979;133:537.

74. Hanna JH, Brady WK, Hill JM, et al: Detection of postmenopausal women at risk for endometrial carcinoma by a progesterone challenge test. Am J Obstet Gynecol 1983;147:872.

75. Henderson BE, Paganini-Hill A, Ross RK: Decreased mortality in users of estrogen replacement therapy. Arch Intern Med 1991;151:75.

76. Henderson BE, Paganini-Hill A, Ross RK: Estrogen replacement therapy and protection from acute myocardial infarction. Am J Obstet Gynecol 1988;159:312.

77. Honjo H, Ogino Y, Naitoh K, et al: In vivo effects by estrone sulfate on the central nervous system: Senile dementia (Alzheimer's type). J Steroid Biochem 1989;34:521.

78. Honjo H, Tamura T, Matsumoto Y, et al: Estrogen as a growth factor to central nervous cells: Estrogen treatment promotes development of acetylcholinesterase: Positive forebrain neurons transplanted in anterior eye chamber. J Steroid Biochem Molec Biol 1992;41:633.

79. Honore LH: Increased incidence of symptomatic cholesterol cholelithiasis in perimenopausal women receiving estrogen replacement therapy. J Reprod Med 1980;25:187.

80. Hortobagyi GN, Hug V, Buzdar AU, et al: Sequential cyclic combined hormonal therapy for metastatic breast cancer. Cancer 1989;64:1002.

81. Hunt K, Vessey M, McPherson K: Long-term surveillance of mortality and cancer incidence in women receiving hormone replacement therapy. Br J Obstet Gynaecol 1987;94:620.

82. Jayo MJ, Weaver DS, Adams MR, et al: Effects on bone of surgical menopause and estrogen therapy with or without progesterone treatment replacement in cynomolgus monkeys. Am J Obstet Gynecol 1990;193:614.

83. Jensen J, Nilas L, Christiansen C: Cyclic changes in serum cholesterol and lipoproteins following different doses of combined postmenopausal replacement therapy. Br J Obstet Gynaecol 1986;93:613.

84. Jick H, Walker AM, Watkins RN, et al: Replacement estrogens and breast cancer. Am J Epidemiol 1980;112:586.

85. Jones B, Russo J: Influence of steroid hormones on the growth fraction of human breast carcinoma. Am J Clin Pathol 1987;88:132.

86. Kakar F, Weiss NS, Strite SA: Noncontraceptive estrogen use and the risk of gallstone disease in women. Am J Public Health 1988;78:564.

87. Kampen DL, Sherwin BB: Estrogen use and verbal memory in healthy postmenopausal women. Obstet Gynecol 1994;83:979.

88. Katahn M: The T-Factor Diet. New York, Bantam Books, Inc. 1993.

89. Kaufman DW, Miller DR, Rosenberg L, et al: Noncontraceptive estrogen use and the risk of breast cancer. JAMA 1984;252:63.

90. Lauritzen C: Ostrogensubstitution in der postmenopause vor und nach behandeltem genital: Und mammakarzinom. Menopause Hormonsubstitution Heute 1993;6:76.

91. Lauritzen C, Meier F: Risks of endometrial and mammary cancer morbidity and mortality in long-term estrogen treatment. In: The Climacteric: An Update. van Herendael H & B, et al (eds.) Lancaster, England: MTP Press, Ltd., 1984;207.

92. Leather AT, Savvas M, Studd JWW: Endometrial histology and bleeding patterns after 8 years of continuous combined estrogen and progestogen therapy. Obstet Gynecol 1991;78:1008.

93. Leonard WG, Doble HP Jr: On the efficacy of a compliance pack in reversing osteoporosis in postmenopausal women. Am J Gynecol Health 1990;4:112.

94. Lind T, Cameron FC, Hunter FM, et al: A prospective controlled trial of six forms of hormone replacement therapy given to postmenopausal women. Br J Obstet Gynaecol 1979;86:1.

95. Lindsay R: Prevention of postmenopausal osteoporosis. Obstet Gynecol Clin N Am 1987;14:63.

96. Lindsay R, Hamet DM, Clark DM: The minimum effective dose of estrogens for prevention of postmenopausal bone loss. Obstet Gynecol 1984;63:759.

97. Lindsay R, Tohme JF: Estrogen treatment of patients with established postmenopausal osteoporosis. Obstet Gynecol 1990;76:290.

98. MacDougall DS: Meeting highlights: Third international symposium on osteoporosis. Drug Ther 1991;21:40.

99. Mack TM, Pike MC, Henderson BE, et al: Estrogens and endometrial cancer in a retirement community. N Engl J Med 1976;294:1262.

100. Magos AL, Brincat M, Studd JWW, et al: Amenorrhea and endometrial atrophy following continuous oral estrogens and progestogen therapy in postmenopausal women. Obstet Gynecol 1985;65:496.

101. Mann JI, Vessey MP, Thorogood M, et al: Myocardial infarction in young women with special reference to oral contraceptive practice. Br Med J 1975;2:241.

102. Mauvais-Jarvis P, Sitruk-Ware R, Kuttem F: Luteal phase defect and breast cancer genesis. Breast Cancer Res Treat 1982;2:139.

103. McFarland KF, Boniface ME, Hornung CA, et al: Risk factors and noncontraceptive estrogen use in women with and without coronary disease. Am Heart J 1989;117:1209.

104. McMichael AJ, Potter JD: Host factors in carcinogenesis: Certain bile-acid metabolic profiles that selectively increase the risk of proximal colon cancer. J Natl Cancer Inst 1985;75:185.

105. Munk-Jensen N, Nielsen SP, Obel EB, et al: Reversal of postmenopausal vertebral bone loss by oestrogen and progestogen: A double-blind placebo controlled study. Br Med J 1988;296:1150.

106. Nabulsi A, Folsom AR, White A, et al: Association of hormone-replacement therapy with various cardiovascular risk factors in postmenopausal women. N Engl J Med 1993;328:1069.

107. Nachtigall LE, Nachtigall RH, Nachtigall RB, et al: Estrogen replacement I: A 10-year prospective study in the relationship to osteoporosis. Obstet Gynecol 1979;53:277.

108. Nachtigall LE, Nachtigall RH, Nachtigall RB, et al: Estrogen replacement II: A prospective study in the relationship to carcinoma and cardiovascular and metabolic problems. Obstet Gynecol 1979;54:74.

109. Nachtigall MJ, Smilen SW, Nachtigall RD, et al: Incidence of breast cancer in a 22-year study of women receiving estrogen-progestin replacement therapy. Obstet Gynecol 1992;80:827.

110. Naessen T, Persson I, Adami H-O, et al: Hormone replacement therapy and the risk for hip fracture. Ann Intern Med 1990;113:95.

111. National Cancer Institute: Surveillance, Epidemiology and End Results (SEER). Bethesda, Biometry Branch of the National Cancer Institute, 1980, p 47.

112. Newcombe PA, Storer BE: Postmenopausal hormone use and risk of large-bowel cancer. J Natl Cancer Inst 1995;87:1067.

113. Notelovitz M: Effect of natural oestrogens on blood pressure and weight in postmenopausal women. S Afr Med J 1975;49:2251.

114. Notelovitz M: Exercise, nutrition, and the coagulation effects of estrogen replacement on cardiovascular health. Obstet Gynecol Clin N Am 1987;14:121.

115. Padwick MC, Pryse-Davies J, Whitehead MI: A simple method for determining the optimal dosage of progestin in postmenopausal women receiving estrogens. N Engl J Med 1986;315:930.

116. Paganini-Hill A, Henderson VW: Estrogen deficiency and risk of Alzheimer's disease in women. Am J Epidemiol 1994;140:256.

117. Paganini-Hill A, Ross RK, Henderson BE: Postmenopausal oestrogen treatment and stroke: A prospective study. Br Med J 1988;297:519.

118. Pallas KG, Holzwarth GJ, Stern MP, et al: The effect of conjugated estrogens on the renin-angiotensin system. J Clin Endocrinol Metab 1977;44:1061.

119. Parker SL, Tong T, Bolden S, Wingo PA, et al: Cancer statistics. CA Cancer J Clin 1997;47:5.

120. Peck WA, Barrett-Conner E, Buckwalter JA, Gambrell RD Jr, et al: Consensus conference: Osteoporosis. JAMA 1984;252:799.

121. Persson I, Yuen J, Bergkvist L, et al: (Letter) Combined estrogen-progestogen replacement and breast cancer risk. Lancet 1992;340:1044.

122. Petitti DB, Perlman JA, Sidney S: Noncontraceptive estrogens and mortality: Long-term follow-up of women in the Walnut Creek study. Obstet Gynecol 1987;70:289.

123. Petranik K, Kable WT, Bewtra C, Gallager JC: (Abstract) Use of progestin challenge test in elderly women: Menopause. J N Am Menopause Soc 1995;2:278.

124. Perez-Jaraiz MD, Revilla M, Alvarez de los Heros JI et al: Prophylaxis of osteoporosis with calcium, estrogens, and/or eelcatonin: Comparative longitudinal study of bone mass. Maturitas 1996;23:327.

125. Prior JC: Progesterone as a bone-trophic hormone. Endocrin Rev 1990;11:368.

126. Punnonen R, Lammintansta R, Erkkda R, et al: Estradiol valerate therapy and the renin-aldosterone system in castrated women. Maturitas 1980;2:91.

127. Riggs BL, Seeman E, Hodgson SF, et al: Effect of the fluoride-calcium regimen on vertebral fracture occurrence in postmenopausal osteoporosis. N Engl J Med 1982;306:446.

128. Riggs BL, Hodgson SF, O'Fallon WM, et al: Effect of the fluoride treatment on the fracture rate in postmenopausal women with osteoporosis. N Engl J Med 1990;322:802.

129. Rosen C, Mallinak N, Cain D et al: A comparison of biochemical markers in monitoring skeletal responses to hormone replacement therapy in early postmenopausal women. J Bone Miner Res 1996;11:5119.

130. Ross RK, Paganini-Hill A, Gerkins VR, et al: A case-control study of menopausal estrogen therapy and breast cancer. JAMA 1980;243:1635.

131. Sarles H, Gerolami A, Cros RC: Diet and cholesterol gallstones: A further study. Digestion 1978;17:128.

132. Sarrel PM: Blood flow. In: Treatment of the Postmenopausal Woman: Basic and Clinical Aspects, RA Lobo, (ed.). New York, Raven Press, 1994, pp 251-262.

133. Sarrel PM: Sexuality in the middle years. Obstet Gynecol Clin N Am 1987;15:49.

134. Schlesselman JJ: Net effect of oral contraceptive use on the risk of cancer of women in the United States. Obstet Gynecol 1995;85:793.

135. Semmens JP, Wagner G: Estrogen deprivation and vaginal function in postmenopausal women. JAMA 1982;248:445.

136. Senie RT, Rosen PP, Rhodes P, et al: Timing of breast cancer excision during the menstrual cycle influences duration of disease-free survival. Ann Intern Med 1991;115:337.

137. Shapiro S, Kelly JP, Rosenberg L, et al: Risk of localized and widespread endometrial cancer in relation to recent and discontinued use of conjugated estrogens. N Engl J Med 1985;313:969.

138. Sherwin BB, Gelfand MM: Differential symptom response to parenteral estrogen and/or androgen administration in the surgical menopause. Am J Obstet Gynecol 1985;151:153.

139. Sillero-Arenas M, Delgado-Rodriguez M, Rodigues-Canteras R, et al: Menopausal hormone replacement therapy and breast cancer: A meta-analysis. Obstet Gynecol 1992;79:286.

140. Smith DC, Prentice R, Thompson DJ, et al: Association of exogenous estrogen and endometrial carcinoma. N Engl J Med 1975;293:1164.

141. Stampfer MJ, Grodstein F: Role of hormone replacement in cardiovascular disease. In: Treatment of the Postmenopausal Woman: Basic and Clinical Aspects, RA Lobo, (ed.). New York, Raven Press, 1994, pp 223-233.

142. Stampfer MJ, Willet WC, Colditz GA, et al: A prospective study of postmenopausal estrogen therapy and coronary heart disease. N Engl J Med 1985;313:1044.

143. Stanczyk FZ, Shoupe D, Nunez V, et al: A randomized comparison of non-oral estradiol delivery in postmenopausal women. Am J Obstet Gynecol 1988;159:1540.

144. Stanford JL, Weiss NS, Voight LF et al: Combined estrogen and progestin hormone replacement therapy in relation to risk of breast cancer in middle-aged women. JAMA 1995;274:137.

145. Steinberg KK, Thacker SB, Smith SJ, et al: A meta-analysis of the effect of estrogen replacement therapy on the risk of breast cancer. JAMA 1991;265:1985.

146. Stoll BA, Parbhoo S: Treatment of menopausal symptoms in breast cancer patients. Lancet 1988;1:1267.

147. Strickland DM, Gambrell RD Jr, Butzin CA, et al: The relationship between breast cancer survival and prior postmenopausal estrogen use. Obstet Gynecol 1992;80:400.

148. Studd J, Magos A: Hormone pellet implantation for the menopause and premenstrual syndrome. Obstet Gynecol Clin N Am 1987;14:229.

149. Studd JWW: The climacteric syndrome. In: Female and Male Climacteric. Serr DM, van Keep PA, Greenblatt RB (eds.) Lancaster, England: MTP Press, Ltd., 1979, p 23.

150. Studd JWW, Collins WP: Oestradiol and testosterone implants in the treatment of psychosexual problems in the postmenopausal woman. Br J Gynaecol 1977;84:314.

151. Sullivan JM, Zwagg RV, Lemp GF, et al: Postmenopausal estrogen use and coronary atherosclerosis. Ann Intern Med 1988;108:358.

152. Tang M-X, Jacobs D, Stern Y et al: Effect of oestrogen during menopause on risk and age at onset of Alzheimer's disease. Lancet 1996;348:429.

153. Thom MH, White PJ, Williams RM, et al: Prevention and treatment of endometrial disease in climacteric women receiving oestrogen therapy. Lancet 1979;2:455.

154. Upton GV: The perimenopause: Physiologic correlates and clinical management. J Reprod Med 1982;27:1.

155. Utian WH: Effect of postmenopausal estrogen therapy on diastolic blood pressure and body weight. Maturitas 1978;1:3.

156. Veronesi U, Luini A, Mariani L, et al: Effect of menstrual phase on surgical treatment of breast cancer. Lancet 1994;343:1545.

157. Voherr H: Oral contraceptives and hormone replacement therapy: Are progestogens and progestins breast mitogens? Am J Obstet Gynecol 1986;155:1140.

158. Wentz WB: Progestin therapy in endometrial hyperplasia. Gynecol Oncol 1974;2:362.

159. Wile AG, Opfell RW, Marileth DA: Hormone replacement therapy in previously treated breast cancer patients. Am J Surg 1993;165:372.

160. Willis DB, Calle EE, Miracle-McMahill HL, et al: Estrogen replacement therapy and risk of fatal breast cancer in a prospective cohort of postmenopausal women in the United States. Cancer Causes and Control 1996;7:449.

161. Wilson PW, Garrison RJ, Willet WC, et al: Postmenopausal estrogen use, cigarette smoking, and cardiovascular morbidity in women over 50: The Framingham Study. N Engl J Med 1985;313:1038.

162. Wingo PA, Layde PM, Lee NC, et al: The risk of breast cancer in postmenopausal women who have used estrogen replacement therapy. JAMA 1987;257:209.

163. Wingo PA, Lee NC, Ory HW et al: Age-specific differences in the relationship between oral contraceptive use and breast cancer. Obstet Gynecol 1991;78:161.

164. Wren BO, Routledge AD: The effect of type and dose of oestrogen on the blood pressure of postmenopausal women. Maturitas 1983;5:135.

165. Writing Group for PEPI Trial: Effects of estrogen or estrogen/progestin regimens on heart disease risk factors in postmenopausal women. JAMA 1995;273:199.

166. Ziel HK, Finkle WD: Increased risk of endometrial carcinoma among users of conjugated estrogens. N Engl J Med 1975;293:1167.

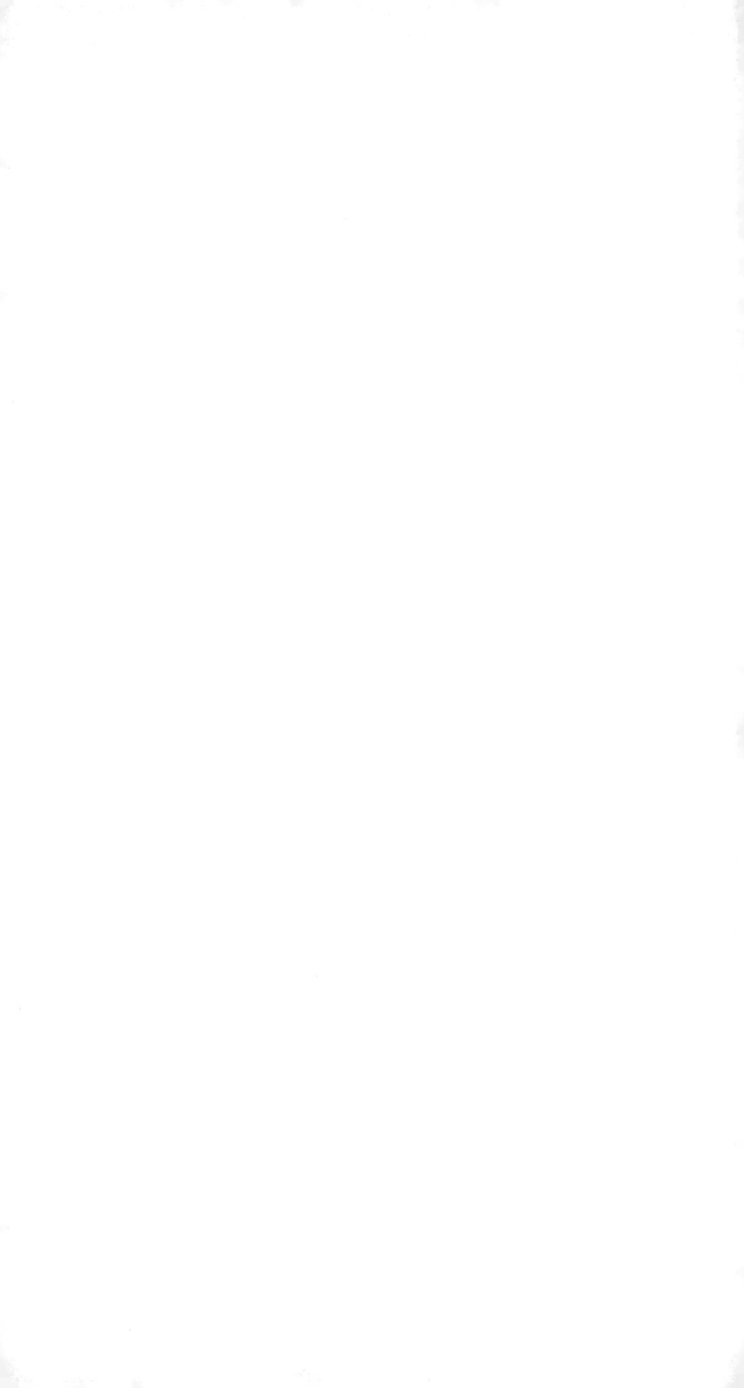